Vegan Nutrition
Endurance Sports

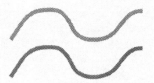

Arnold Wiegand

Vegan + Sports

Vegan Nutrition and Endurance Sports

Wiegand, Arnold:
Vegan + Sports
Vegan Nutrition and Endurance Sports
ISBN 3-00-017853-8

Copyright © January 2006   by   Arnold Wiegand
Mainblick 5
65779 Kelkheim
Germany

Published by:
Arnold Wiegand, Mainblick 5, 65779 Kelkheim - Germany

Original Title: Vegan + Sport
              Vegane Ernährung und Ausdauersport
              ISBN 3-8334-4129-1

Translated from the German by:
              Charles Frantz
              1405 Terrace Drive, Suite 23
              St Paul, MN 55113 USA
              http://home.comcast.net/~jwgoethe/

ISBN 3-00-017853-8

Important Note

The recommendations in this book have been carefully tested by the author. The book does not replace personal perception. The reader is required to convince himself/herself of its effectiveness in his/her personal situation. Sometimes small changes are necessary in training or diet.

This book is not intended to be a replacement for medical advice, or for seeing a doctor. Every reader is responsible for his/her own actions. Therefore, all information in this book is provided without the guarantee of the author.
The author cannot be held responsible for personal injuries, property damage or financial losses.

A vegan diet (that is, the non-consumption of all animal products) is not automatically healthy. Vegan nutrition will not prevent or cure every disease. Optimal results can only be achieved when one pays attention to the quantity and quality of one's diet, taking into consideration one's personal situation.
A vegan diet can be an important factor in maintaining good health.
Additionally, there are other factors which influence health, such as stress, lifestyle, physical exercise (sports), etc.

In spite of careful examination of content the author assumes no responsibility for the contents of internet pages or web sites which are mentioned in the book. The web site creators are solely responsible for the content of their sites. They only serve to inform the reader. They cannot be relied upon by the reader to be correct, complete or current.
The above disclaimers shall also apply to the translator.

Additional and current information about

Vegan Nutrition and Endurance Sports

can be found at

    www.vegan-sports.de

    e-mail@vegan-sports.de

Contents

Nutrition

Endurance Sports

Acknowledgments

In recent years I have experienced many changes and positive personal developments.

I would like to take this opportunity to thank the people who have supported and encouraged me in my development.
A special "thank you" to Irisia, for it was her support that made it possible to lay the groundwork for this book.

I also thank my wife for the photos and her support in the creation of this book.

Foreword

Why have I written this book?

I decided to begin a vegan diet (that is, consuming no animal products whatsoever) in the spring of 2003.

At the same time I began marathon training. I felt a great need for information, due both to an insecure feeling and a lack of knowledge.
I obtained the knowledge from a great variety of sources, went over it carefully and internalized that which seemed helpful.

Despite thorough research, I was unable to locate a single source in which vegan nutrition and endurance sports were covered. I was particularly interested in marathon swimming and long-distance running as well as the Ironman Triathlon.
There was just as little detailed background information or reports from personal experience of vegan endurance athletes.

This book will serve as a guide for those who are dealing with such questions as:

"What advantages can a vegan diet and endurance sports afford me?"

"Is a vegan diet compatible with endurance sports?"

"What are the necessary steps to achieve my fitness goals, and what do I have to pay the most attention to?"

To answer a few questions in advance:

Yes -- It is possible to acquire the knowledge needed for a healthy vegan diet and to learn the basics of endurance sports in a short period of time.

Yes -- It is possible to be a vegan and to successfully participate in endurance sports.

Yes -- There are well--known athletes, both men and women, who are vegans.

Yes -- It is possible to maintain good health with the appropriate nourishment.

Yes -- It is possible to reach one's ideal weight and to maintain it.

My training recommendations are tailored to suit both those who are just learning an endurance sport (such as running) as well as those who wish to train for an ultra-marathon.

This book is based on both knowledge and experience. It will make starting easier and save time for the reader, for further research will not be necessary.
I have personally tested all of the training and diet suggestions for their effectiveness.

In some parts of the book I intentionally speak in only general terms.

This is because I want to encourage the reader to internalize the information in a personal way, and to take that which fits his/her own situation.

What good does a fantastic training plan for a marathon consisting of 4 units do, if someone doesn't have time for 4 units?

For this reason, I show how you can create your own training plan, and tell you what to remember to include in it.

Vegan Recipes for Endurance Athletes will be published as a separate book in early 2006.

I am always available for personal consultation.

I offer seminars on vegan nutrition and endurance sports for novice as well as elite athletes in Germany, Austria and Switzerland.
You only need to ask me, and I am prepared to do the same thing in other locations such as North America and Great Britain.

I can also coach you personally.

In the seminars and coaching I go into the technical aspects of this book more deeply and expand on them. In addition, special conditioning exercises are taught. These help with flexibility and body posture, among other things.

In the seminars, all participants are coached in these areas:

-- vegan nutrition

-- proper running and swimming

-- personal training regimen

-- mental fitness

-- conditioning / upper body exercises

A word about mental fitness -- here I will help you to overcome mental blocks, poor behavioral models, self-defeating attitudes, and much more.

To find out dates and times of seminars and/or obtain the most current information, go to **www.vegan-sports.de**

Please e-mail me personally at **e-mail@vegan-sports.de** if you have any questions or comments.

14

About Myself

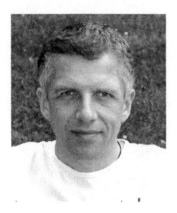

Born in 1963, married, 2 children

Higher education: Coursework in various methods for the purpose of promoting personal growth in myself and others.
(For example, 2 year degree in Psychological Counseling, 2 year degree in Systematic Supervision and Coaching, studied different communications models, among others, NLP.)

Professional Experience (in part)
  7 years   Personnel Manager
  3 years   Held seminars for and coached executives and
            managers, Taught Team Development

How it all began . . .

and where it has led to so far . . .

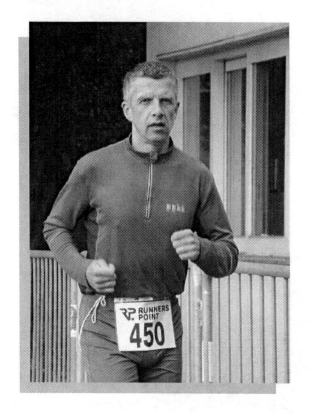

Right before the finish -- 162k (101 miles)

24 hour long-distance race   Basel, 2005

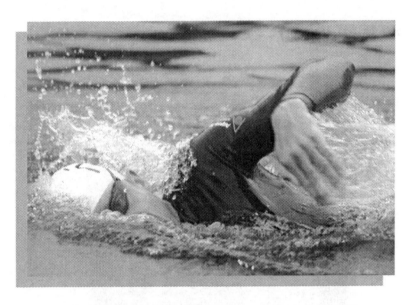

Soon I will have swum 26.4k non-stop . . . (9:57)
Lake Zurich Swim, 2005

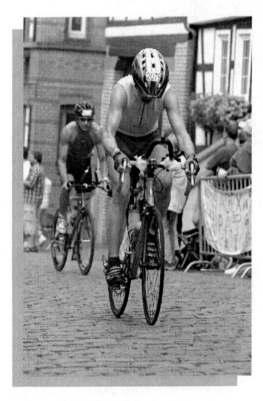

My first Triathlon

Ironman -
Frankfurt, 2005
11:56

Swimming   3.8k
Cycling   180k
Running   42.2k

© ASI Photo
www.asiphoto.net

Sports – My History

Starting at age 20, I ran a half-marathon three years in a row. Because I hadn't trained enough, I found the last one to be quite difficult.

For 15 years after that I did virtually nothing when it came to endurance sports.
Every two months or so I would swim one kilometer, and every two weeks I ran just three kilometers.

When I hit 40 (in 2003), I began to deal with my attitudes and behavior very intensively, though recognizing that these traits were the result of my upbringing and societal influences.
In many cases I decided that a major change was called for. Apparently this process had an effect on my athletic ambitions.

My job took me to another city where I began running three or four times a week. At the beginning 10k (6 miles) a day, and a few weeks later I was up to 15k.
Then I had a brilliant insight: "In autumn there will be a half-marathon here -- maybe I could give it a whirl."

I looked on the internet for training regimens, and read runners' reports of their personal experiences.

Here I stumbled upon the information that in nearby Frankfurt there is a marathon every year. I was beaming on the inside, and I just knew I would take part.
I had no idea how I could perform on this level, but there were still a few months to get ready ... .
In the meantime I swam 5-7k once each week.

I took off 15 kilograms (= 33 pounds) of weight (even though I was putting on muscle) in the several months preceding the marathon.

I discovered that I now weighed the same as I did when I was only 19 years old, 75 kilograms (165 lbs).

I have managed to maintain this weight and the good feeling that came with it ever since. (My weight only varies very slightly +/- 1kg, which is the result of differing training regimens).

I participated in the Frankfurt marathon in October of 2003, arriving at the finish line after 4 hours and 12 minutes.

Following this, I informed myself further concerning long-distance running.

I came upon information and personal experiences in 100 km (62 miles) races. I had no idea how I could make this become reality for myself nor even why I wanted to do it, but was filled with joy when I thought "I'll do it next spring!"

Competitions 2004

In December of 2003 I began training for a 100k race, following a training schedule. Part of the plan was to participate in a marathon, in order to test my form.

April 25, 2004   Weiltal, 63k Marathon

So I registered for the Weiltal Marathon. Then the idea occurred to me, "Why should I just run the marathon, when I am training for a much longer distance?"
I decided to run from home to the start of the marathon (21k with one big hill after another).

My planning was right on target: I got to the starting line with ten minutes to spare, handed over my backpack with a change of clothes in it, and lined up with the other participants.
And that's how it began – my first Ultra-marathon.

I ran the marathon in 4:08. Altogether I had run 63 kilometers in six hours and twenty minutes.

In order to test my reserve energy supply, I didn't accept any nourishment during the race other than a lot of water.
But after I crossed the finish line, I let myself have all the bananas and apples I could wolf down.

I came back on the train, and ran home easily, feeling loose. I felt in top form and knew I could handle the 100k race.

May 22, 2004   Odensee/Stige,
**   Long-distance run – 100k**

Four weeks after the first ultra-run the time had come: I had decided to participate in the 100k race in Odensee/Stige (Denmark).
It is a flat course -- ten kilometers per lap.

Everything went splendidly up to the 70th kilometer (6 hrs and 49 min), but then an ice cold wind blew in some hard rain. Although I wore a thin plastic poncho, my arms and legs were wet and ice cold, and this took its toll on performance and motivation.

While leaving the next day I became aware that I had exceeded my personal limits in this race. Thus, a new period was about to begin … .

In reading this, one could gain the impression that I had taken part in competitions more or less effortlessly. To an extent, that is correct.

But I have had other experiences:

August 8, 2004   Lake Zurich, Swimming – 16k

In the summer of 2004 I took part in the Lake Zurich Swim (26.4k). In training I swam 30k per week for several weeks, 14k each time in the space of a week in a training sequence.

And then: In the competition I was over one hour slower over the first 16 kilometers than I had been in training (compared to the 14k in training), and went over the allotted time for this segment.

Surely the reason was a mental problem, for I was physically fit, but inside I somehow didn't have enough drive to attain a higher speed.

But it was completely different in 2005!

Note: Based on my experience in 2005 I can say that one reason for the failure lay in the fact that I hadn't eaten anything during the 16k stretch, and didn't notice how my performance began to slip. This was only one aspect, though, for in training (2 x 14k) I hadn't taken any nourishment either, and despite this was one hour faster (compared to the 16k).

October 2, 2004   Mulhouse, 24 Hour Run

After having had a very good experience in spring with the 100k run, I was confident that I could successfully participate in a 24 hour run. The race took place in an inner city park. The course was flat, and consisted of asphalt and solid fine gravel.

In the race something strange happened (compared with my experience in Lake Zurich two months prior):
At kilometer 101 tendon pain in the left instep forced me to drop out of the competition.

I had never felt pain in this area, and I ran in the same running shoes that I had worn for a few hundred miles in training.
After that I also wore the same shoes without experiencing any problems.

Since then I haven't had this problem, not even with the very same running shoes.

October 21, 2004   Landau, Swimming – 20.4k

Two weeks after these two unsatisfying experiences I took part in a twelve hour swimming race. The challenge was that the competition was to take place during the night (8:00 pm to 8:00 am).
I really felt good, though my performance suffered at night due to tiredness and lowered metabolism.
Yet I successfully completed my first nighttime competition.

Competitions 2005

March 6, 2005   Zurich, Swimming – 26.1k

In March of 2005 I took part in the twelve hour swim in Zurich, Switzerland. After eight hours I began to experience pain in the bicep tendons, and I had to slow down.
Although I had trained less than in the previous year, I swam 26.1 kilometers.

**May 7, 2005   Basel, 24 Hour Run – 162k
                    (101 miles)**

I had long been fascinated by a 24 hour race, so I registered for the competition in Basel, Switzerland.
The course turned out to be a tough nut to crack -- 24 hours on a flat, round course, 1,140 meters, on asphalt.

This was already demanding enough, but heavy rain showers for eight hours and a strong wind made it even tougher.
During the night the temperature went down to five degrees Celsius (that would be 41 degrees in the U.S.).
Altogether 63 runners from nine countries started the race. I finished 14th among the 36 male finishers, having run 162k.
The winner ran 225k.
There was another vegan in the race (he ran 155k).

At the 30 kilometer mark I began to notice the tendons in my feet. I was thinking: It can't be true, this problem making itself known so soon?
I changed shoes at 50k, and after that, all went splendidly.

After three hours I accepted some tomatoes and cucumbers. After 50 kilometers I had some warm millet, and then again at kilometer 100 and also 130.

Owing to the low temperature I drank mostly warm water.

After over 100 kilometers I allowed myself to sleep in a tent for two and a half hours. To my surprise my legs had no difficulty in getting started again and I felt really fit.

At some point the sun came up and I thought to myself, "Already another marathon run and I have achieved my goal".

I had pictured myself running over 160 kilometers in the race. And that is precisely what happened. But I had two problems to deal with beginning at kilometer 150: the tendons on the instep and a large blister on the ball of my right foot.

During the eight weeks preceding the run I ran every Saturday (6 x 45k and 2 x 50k).

My training regimen: In 2005 I was doing a weekly average of 65 kilometers. The weekly average during the last two months before the 24 hour race was 75k. The peak was 2 x 95k.

But no more than that.

It was actually far too little (I had done a lot more running to prepare for the first 100k race). But I have developed my own training style, and I had the feeling that it was quite sufficient.

The next day I stepped onto the scale, and it read 75kg, the same as it had before the race.

And that was exactly how I felt, too: I had the feeling that I had lost no physical substances, but rather, that the run had strengthened me both mentally and physically.

July 10, 2005   Frankfurt, Ironman Triathlon 11:56

I had always admired triathletes for their ability to develop a training regimen which prepared them for three disciplines by the day of the competition.

The demands are unreal -- especially in the longest triathlon, the Ironman.

When I registered for the competition in October 2004, I just knew I would be fit in 2005. But I had very little cycling experience and didn't even own a racing bicycle.
I didn't buy one until six months before the race. Would this provide enough time to get ready to ride a bicycle competitively?

This is how the race went:

-- Swimming 3.8k 1:06

   ... and this after having been kicked in the chin twice -- once at the mass start and another time at a turn.
   So I swam the rest of the way more defensively. In any event, I achieved a good time for my purposes.

-- Cycling 180k   5:46

   Everything went perfectly. I averaged 31 kilometers per hour, even though I had only owned a racing bike for six months.

-- Running 42.2k   4:40

   This part went miserably. After one kilometer I had to walk for a while. I thought that things would get better, but this didn't happen. I had eaten enough and had no complaints, but where had my energy gone?

Conclusion? The balance of the experience had been gratifying. Anyway, it was my first triathlon.

Taking part in a competition in the presence of several hundred thousand spectators had been very special.

July 24, 2005   Lake Zurich,
**   Marathon Swim – 26.4 Kilometers 9:57**

The past year's failure proved to be a burden on me both in training and in the race itself. I trained less and introduced more variations into my regimen.

When I registered for the event I decided to swim in a neoprene suit (1 mm).
The water temperature was at 20 degrees Celsius (= 68 degrees Fahrenheit).
The swimmers who didn't wear a protective suit had allowed themselves to put on a little fat for protection against hypothermia.

Every swimmer was accompanied by a boat. I had made arrangements for millet to be given to me every hour for an energy supply. This was to enable me to maintain my swimming speed (altogether I ate about one kilogram of millet = 2.2 pounds).
Eating was very uncomfortable, though, using one hand to eat and the other to paddle so that I would remain above water.
Holding onto the boat would have led to disqualification.

It went along like this, until I reached kilometer 14 (after five hours and eight minutes). Gradually I became aware of irritations in my bicep tendons. But this was so subtle that I didn't have to slow down.

In the course of swimming I often got cramps in a calf, and once in the thigh as well. Despite the pain I merely kept swimming, varying my movements a little. Fortunately this was sufficient to stop the cramps after a minute or two.

In these situations I found it helpful to concentrate on just two things: the distance to the escort boat and my next arm stroke. I paid no attention to the scenery, the distance I had come or had yet to go, or other thoughts.

Another swimmer was of the opinion that the cause of the cramps was probably that I only breathe on the left side, causing an asymmetry in the body.

I had no calf cramps during the last two hours of the swim.

I swam at a fairly regular pace, needing four hours and 57 minutes for the remaining 12.4k. This despite the fact that the waves got pretty big for a lake in the last three hours.

I reached the finish after nine hours and 57 minutes. I was (and still am) very satisfied with the time, above all because I had had very little experience over long distances.

On the way home I looked down at Lake Zurich from a mountain. I could only see half of the lake, but that was enough to comprehend what a great distance I had swum non-stop, and that I had significantly extended previous mental and physical limits.

August 20, 2005   Interlaken, Inferno-Triathlon

For my second triathlon I decided on one of the toughest triathlon competitions.

Distances and Conditions:
-- Swimming 3.1k   Water temperature 17 degrees Celsius (62F)
-- Cycling 92k   2,145 meter climb
-- Mountain bike 30k 1,180 meter climb
-- Running 25k   2,175 meter climb

I required 1:06 for the swim and changeover and was in 51st place.
Things went pretty well on the racing bicycle, although I did have to get off and push the bicycle as I approached the last summit. I had used a lot of energy in riding up the mountain. There were no flat places at all, only climbs.

Then came the mountain bike segment. It rained hard beginning right at the changeover and it never stopped all day long. The climbing began right away, no rest all the way to the summit.

As the path led to the top my performance reserves were drastically reduced. I had to push the bike for an unconscionable amount of time. It was small consolation that other participants were having the same experience.
I had no pains and my mood was good, but the prior climbs had made quite a dent in my supply of reserve energy.

I reached the changeover zone to running right before the cut-off. If I had changed clothes as fast as lightning I might have left the zone on time.
But it was clear to me that I wouldn't be able to make the required running times for each segment.
I would have still been good for a run on level ground, but another 25k on a climb of 2,175 meters?
To be perfectly honest, I had conquered 3,300 meters of climbing, but ended my participation here.

Why was that?

-- Aren't mountain races and I the best of friends?
-- Were the distances and conditions too demanding for my fitness level at the time?
-- Didn't I allow enough time to regenerate after the Ironman and the Lake Zurich swim two weeks later?

Competitions 2006

Information concerning future races will be published on the Internet at **www.vegan-sports.de**

These are my plans so far for 2006:

Long-distance running: 24 hour race

Swimming: Crossing the Baltic Sea 21-25k (current)
www.beltquerung.de

Triathlon: Ironman-Frankfurt

What motivates me to realize such athletic accomplishments?

During the last two years I discovered a talent that had lain dormant in me for decades. I wasn't aware of it, and never took advantage of it.
I have decided to make use of this ability, without striving for any particular kind of athletic development, (at least at the beginning), or knowing where this decision might lead me.

Diet – My Past

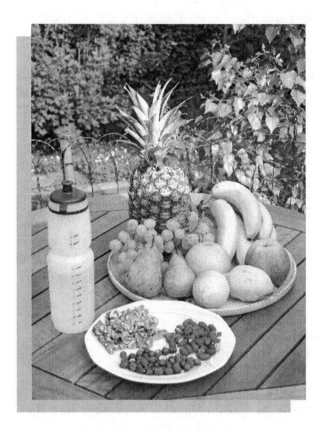

The decision (at age 26) to start a vegetarian diet was actually not a decision in the true sense of the word. I simply no longer had a desire to eat meat or fish. And it stayed like that for 13 years.

In the spring of 2003 I made the decision to immediately begin a vegan diet.

I noticed that the food set very well with me, was better and more rapidly digested, and thus that more energy was available to me.

One example: I had enjoyed the taste of cheese very much, and I had eaten it regularly. After these meals, I noticed a certain heaviness in my stomach, which I had in the past always blamed on the fact that I had eaten too much.
Since I have been eating vegan I can state definitively that the problem wasn't the amount, but rather that the cheese was a burden on my body (and thus cost me energy).

Whatever the reason might have been, I was neither willing to nor able to pay attention to my body's signals.
This has changed drastically since making the switch to a vegan diet.
Through intensive endurance sports I am made aware of which foods are good for me and/or which I require at the moment.
Vegan nourishment and endurance training were and are a perfect match for me.

The Basis of my Thinking

As I became concerned with the topic of nutrition and ultra-marathon/endurance sports I quickly became aware that there are a variety of points of view and serious prejudices.

A vegan/vegetarian diet is especially inundated with prejudices:

-- "Vegetarians are without energy, are worn-out quickly, emaciated, have no endurance ..."

-- "Meat contains the greatest amount of protein."
    False: Meat contains about 20% protein.
             Beans, lentils, ... about 22-30% protein.
             Soy exceeds this with about 39%.

-- "Milk has the highest amount of calcium."
    False: The calcium content of a few foods
             in mg per 100 grams --

    Soybeans   257
    Kale   230
    Nuts   225-234
    Milk   120
    Broccoli   113

When I was 28 I rode the streetcar in Frankfurt, carrying two shopping bags full of vegetables. A nice and short dialog developed with a female senior citizen:
    Well, you eat a lot of vegetables!
        Yes, I'm a vegetarian.
    But you don't look like one at all.

Apparently some people think of vegetarians as being emaciated and having a sunken face.

In spite of the many different prejudices, I have the impression that vegetarians are experiencing greater acceptance.

Vegans are still looked upon as if they came from a different planet. If a vegetarian supposedly creeps through life listlessly and without energy, then a vegan must be in the last stage of malnourishment.

A few questions which I encountered after switching to a vegan diet will elucidate this further:

-- Where do you get your protein from?
   Animal protein is better than plant protein!
-- Vegan nutrition is unhealthy!
-- You aren't getting enough vitamins!

> **Typically, these questions are asked by precisely those persons who are overweight, suffer from a lack of exercise, and pay little attention to quality, highly nutritious foods.**
>
> **And who have to deal with all sorts of nutrition-related physical ailments!**

When I tell people that I am both a vegan and an endurance athlete, these prejudices crumble into small parts.

Suddenly there are no arguments to be heard when I begin to talk about 100k races, 12 hour swims, a 24 hour marathon or the Ironman triathlon.

If I hadn't chosen the most optimal diet for myself, I wouldn't have been capable of such athletic performance, especially not of enhancing performance in such a short period of time.

At age 40 I ran the first marathon, six months later I ran 100k in 10:33, and twelve months after that I ran 162k (101 miles) in a 24 hour competition.

Since I have been eating vegan, I feel a lot more energetic and my energy is quickly replenished.

I attribute this to the end products of metabolism being excreted more quickly and fewer burdensome substances being ingested (feed additives and pharmaceuticals used in raising animals, ingredients such as refined sugar or preservatives in the normal foods, purine).

That is one of the reasons why my body absorbs the nutrients better.

The fact is that normal food is in the digestive tract at least twice as long.

And that presents, for example, the danger of putrefaction or flatulence. To put it concretely, it costs the body energy and consequently a person doesn't feel well.

I am of the opinion that anyone (especially the endurance athlete) who does not concern himself/herself intensively with diet, energy provision and metabolism will quite quickly find himself/herself in an undernourished state, regardless of whether it is the usual food or a vegan diet.

Vegan nutrition is not automatically healthy and the optimal diet. It is important to pay attention to the body's signals in one's own actual situation, and to the food that is called for.

As a result of my previous enculturation I felt insecure about the change to a vegan diet, and I informed myself about the nutritional ingredients, their absorption into the body and what an endurance athlete requires.

And it is precisely that which is noteworthy: Although I had decided upon a qualitatively better and more healthy diet, I wanted to be better informed.

Actually this would have been much more important before the switch. And when one takes a look at all of the maladies which can be traced back to diet, it would be sensible for everyone to deal intensively with questions of nourishment.

Even the running magazines are increasingly dealing with the topic of the connection between diet and endurance sports:

"The way of compensating for lack of movement and its results is almost too simple: exercise – fast walking or running.
The alternative to improper nutrition is only simple on first glance: eat properly. But what does properly mean? Because diet is determined by an overweight market, misinformation is the order of the day as a result of business interests. Maintaining good health remains an information problem."

Source: 1

The Vegan Way of Life

In addition to my physical well-being, I perceive vegan nourishment to be a matter of responsibility to myself, animals and the environment. For this reason I have chosen, quite apart from diet, to refrain from using products which contain animal parts.

By what right are pet animals (which are endlessly coddled and petted) differentiated from non-domestic animals? Pets are comprehensively protected. Practically everything is denied other animals.

A few examples (the list could unfortunately be effortlessly expanded):

By what right may, for example, 45 million male chicks be killed in Germany -- only because they don't lay any eggs for breakfast? The male chicks are gassed immediately after hatching, or ground alive into puree.
That is the reality -- even in 2005.
One who buys eggs accepts this state of affairs consciously or subconsciously.

Source: **2**

Not so very long ago the oceans still appeared to be an inexhaustible source of fish and other marine life. That has changed drastically. More and more kinds of fish are being threatened with extinction.
This affects above all the fishing industry. The consequences can hardly be assessed.

Catch quotas and prohibitions have not been sufficient to rebuild the threatened species for the longest time, for over-fishing disturbs the balance of the entire ecosystem.

Ocean floor dragging nets are destroying the bottom of the ocean completely. When this method is used, all kinds of marine life are collected.

The fishing industry simply accepts the fact that for one sole fish, over 10 kilograms of unwanted catch are killed and thrown overboard.

Fish suffer when they are speared alive, tossed around, squashed or mutilated, and often they are left to die a slow and painful death by asphyxiation.

Source: 3

For what reason is it viewed as normal and tolerated that lobsters are boiled alive? Lobsters possess a nervous system and experience a great deal of pain for a long time while they are being cooked. They are only unable to express this pain in a way that people can recognize it.

Just like other vertebrates, including humans, fish are equipped with a highly developed system which can protect them from severe pain -- pain that informs them that their life could be in danger, when they are severely impaired by a physical injury, say by a large predator.

This system releases substances similar to opium (encephalin and endorphins) as soon as an animal is injured … .

The existence of this pain numbing opium system implies that an ability to feel pain must be present. Otherwise, it wouldn't make any sense that such a system developed in animals at all.

Source: 4

Australia produces 30 percent of the world's wool. The most commonly bred sheep there are the merinos, which were bred to have skin with many folds, so that the wool yield per animal will be greater. This unnaturally large amount of wool leads to many sheep collapsing during the hot months and dying of heat stroke. In addition, moisture and urine collect in the skin folds. Flies are attracted by the moisture and lay their eggs in these folds, and the larvae which hatch can consume the sheep alive.

In the attempt to prevent this, the Australian ranchers perform a barbaric operation on the animals -- "mulesing".

In this process they cut away -- without any anesthesia -- pieces of flesh as large as dinner plates from the area around the tail. In doing so they hope to cause an uncreased, scarred surface to form which no longer serves as a place for fly eggs to be laid.

But ironically, these large, bloody wounds are often attacked by flies before they can heal.

Source/Note:

PETA (www.peta.de www.peta.org) is presently negotiating an agreement with the Australian wool industry. But it would not agree to refrain from mulesing, although pain-killers would be used.

Thus, the suffering of the sheep would merely be eased, and not prevented.

How did I make the change to the vegan diet and way of life?

I changed my diet completely overnight. Now, instead of being a vegetarian, I was a vegan. With no exceptions, ifs, ands or buts.

I replaced some clothing, shoes and furniture immediately, and some in the course of the past years. I will make more replacements as items wear out.
Often it is not a financial question, but rather one of personal taste or where the new items can be had in the case of things that are not so common.

Alternatives

It is not necessary to produce wrist watches, footballs, upholstery, belts, coats, shoes nor anything else from leather.
There are many alternative materials, for example cotton, linen, rubber, ramie, sailcloth and synthetic materials. These are less expensive and don't contribute toward mass slaughtering for meat or the wild hunt for animals with wonderful fur.
It is not a sacrifice to wear leather-free articles of clothing, for more and more manufacturers are already producing alternative goods which are not only attractive but also durable.

Refraining from the use of any and all animal products in one's diet, dress or home furnishings shows respect for the animals as that, which they are:
Creatures with their own value and own feelings -- not just the objects of human exploitation and capriciousness.

Vegan Athletes

Here are just a few of the most famous athletes who eat a vegan diet:

Martina Navratilova
> World class tennis pro for over 20 years

Carl Lewis
> 9 Olympic gold medals

Dr. Ruth Heidrich
> World class Ironwoman
> Winner of several Ironman competitions

Brendan Brazier
> Professional Triathlete

Scott Jurek
> World class Ultra-marathon runner
> Winner: Badwater 135 mile race and
> 7 times Western States 100 mile race

The Vegan Diet and Lifestyle

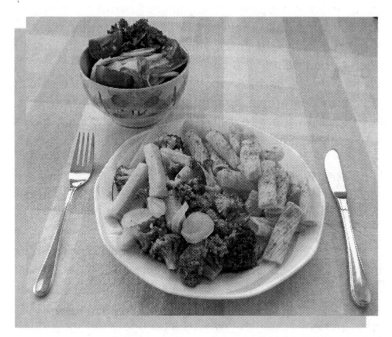

For Starters: Cucumbers, Tomatoes, Herbs, Vegan Salad Dressing, Salt
Main Dish: Noodles, Zucchini, Onions, Broccoli, Curry, Spices

What does "vegan" mean?

First off, the word is properly pronounced "veegan" in English. As is the case with every lifestyle, the vegan way of life is personally defined by everyone who has decided on it.

All vegans have in common avoiding animal foods such as meat, fish, milk, eggs and honey.

Vegans who are ethically motivated refuse not only animal food products, but they also refrain, insofar as it is possible, from using other products whose manufacture causes animals to suffer (for example, woolen clothing, leather and silk).

Source: 5

Important Note:

Apparently the vegan diet is viewed with many prejudices. Some non-vegans are of the opinion that people following the vegan way of life are fundamentally malnourished. On the other hand, some vegans believe that the nourishment they take is practically guaranteed to be healthy and correct.
Research has shown both viewpoints to be wrong. A well-planned vegan diet provides ample amounts of all essential nutrients, but one has to stick to the generally recognized nutritional guidelines in order to achieve a healthy diet.

There is no strictly defined typical vegan nourishment, and it is the responsibility of every individual to take in the nutrients necessary for his/her current situation in life.

What I have written in this book regarding vegan (sports) nutrition has primarily to do with the diet I have put together to suit my personal needs.
As everyone is living in a different situation, has a different past diet, and is pursuing his/her own athletic goals, an individual plan is not only sensible but also necessary.

This is not peculiar to vegan nutrition, but rather should be normal nutritional behavior.

You can read about the avoidance of healthy nutrition and/or the neglect of further education in the area of diet in, for example

The 2004 Nutritional Report of the German Federal Government

as follows:

The German Diet: too much, too sweet, too fatty

... The report shows: The Germans continue to consume too many calories. The result: More than 65% of the men and 55% of the women are overweight. And the numbers are increasing all the time.
Improper nutrition and excess weight lead to diseases caused by diet, which are already responsible for about two thirds of all deaths ...

... People are eating more vegetables and fruit than before. We are taking care of two thirds of our daily energy requirement with plant foods. But with an average of 150 grams per day we are still far from reaching the 400 grams of fruit and vegetables per day that the World Health Organization recommends ...

... If everyone consumed this amount the risk of cancer could be lowered by 20 percent in women and as much as 30 percent in men. "This should actually persuade everyone", Federal Consumer Minister Künast emphasizes ...

... The frequency of and seriousness of overweight and adiposis (fat addiction, obesity) is increasing alarmingly, not only in adults, but also in children and adolescents. 10 to 15 percent of elementary school children are already overweight, with this trend on the increase ...

Source: 6 Ernährungsbericht 2004 der Bundesregierung

How good is the diet of athletes?

The Rhine/Ruhr Olympic Training Center, together with the Niederrhein Technical University, investigated the dietary habits of 40 performance and recreational athletes.

The results clearly reveal that both groups of athletes did not succeed in covering their needs for vitamins, minerals and trace elements.

Only in isolated cases did the athletes get the amounts of the 21 researched nutrients which the German Dietary Association recommends.

Performance athletes were better nourished than the recreational athletes on the average, but they were only getting half (at the most) of the recommended daily requirement of many vitamins. Even the classic sport vitamins were found to be insufficient.

Five servings of fruit and vegetables per day, as has been recommended for years do not represent the usual diet.

Other research by the Olympic Centers in Frankfurt and Stuttgart painted a similar picture.

Obviously many athletes are overtaxed by the recommendations for healthy nutrition due to their hectic day.

Source: 7

My observations on the athletes I know

People usually know the significance, necessity and effects of a healthy diet.

In **general** inquiries they mention again and again "that one should orient oneself to that and regularly eat fruit and vegetables".

In **targeted** inquiries we become aware that fruit and vegetables are consumed only in small portions and not frequently enough. Only when we ask further questions are the unhealthy eating habits mentioned.

It only becomes apparent that most people just have superficial knowledge and that implementation is done half-heartedly when we ask for **detailed knowledge** like, for example:
-- the contents of nuts,
-- the meaning of Omega-3 fatty acids,
-- the effects of poor diet on health
   (heart and circulatory diseases, type 2 diabetes, etc.), or
-- the occurrence and effect of minerals present in fruit and
   vegetables.

This is not surprising at all. How should people know these things? Even in the education of medical doctors nutrition science has almost no place (only within the framework of personal initiative or further education in this specialty).

When it is a little more difficult or time consuming to prepare healthy food, for example at work, while traveling, or after work, compromises are quickly made -- "On Sunday I will eat something healthy!".

Information regarding a healthy (sports) diet is available and easily obtainable.

But it must be sought out in a great variety of sources, and this uses up valuable time and requires effort. In addition, it is a challenge to sort out intentionally incorrect or incomplete information.

In one magazine the importance of doing without nuts (especially walnuts) was mentioned as an example of calorie-conscious eating. There was no mention of the composition of nuts and its significance; for example, the high concentrations of vitamins and minerals, and, in the case of walnuts, the extremely important Omega-3 fatty acids.

How does your diet stack up?

I advise you to be honest in your self-appraisal.

No excuses, justifications or explanations.

Do take the time now, and make a written record of the present state of your eating behavior. For just one week, write down what and how much you drink and eat. This will best be done in the evening.

	Beverages Which?	Beverages How much?	Food What?	Food How much?
Monday -- Breakfast -- Snack -- Lunch -- Snack -- Dinner -- Evening				
Tuesday				
Wednesday				
Thursday				
Friday				
Saturday				
Sunday				

When you are finished reading this book, take a look at your entries in the table above at your leisure, and check to see whether and in what area a correction is appropriate.

-- How does your intake of the basic nutritional substances look (protein, carbohydrates and fats?)

-- How does your intake of vital nutrients look (vitamins, minerals, trace elements ...)

-- What about fluids?

-- Do you have complaints that can be traced back to your diet, or that could be alleviated by means of optimized nourishment?

Make up a plan -- insofar as some aspect could be improved upon, or that you would like to optimize.

Depending upon your personal situation, it could make sense to begin with small steps (for example, substituting two apples in the morning for those two chocolate bars), or you may prefer to make a complete change in diet.

Both approaches have advantages and disadvantages.

The deciding factors are motivation and imagination, along with flexibility in implementing the new diet.

Existing reservations and outdated viewpoints

A few decades ago doctors were still occupied with making vegetarians aware of the many supposed shortcomings of their diet.
Thus the medical research of meat-eating scientists was very intensively concerned with all possible nutrients.

This led to vegetarianism having been much better researched in many matters of detail than the usual meat-oriented diet, which one assumed to be a given.

As it began to be noticed that a vegetarian diet was more effective in providing vitamins and other vital nutrients than a non-vegetarian lifestyle, scientists began in the nineties to study the health advantages of this diet.
During this time period ca. 75 scientific articles were published on this topic per year.

The official teaching, which had long warned people against taking up a vegetarian diet (and especially a vegan one), was brought increasingly into question through these more recent studies.
Yet one could always claim that not enough was known about this subject and that therefore further studies were necessary, before one could be certain that vegetarian nutrition is actually healthy.

Obviously the fact that almost all of the scientists were carnivores and were still hoping that their diet was the better one played a role in delaying the research.

Human Physiology

According to statements from biologists and anthropologists, who study our anatomy and evolution, humans are plant eaters, and are not particularly suited to the consumption of meat.

Although people today take in a great variety of plant and animal foodstuffs, which gave us the nickname "omnivores", from an anatomical standpoint we remain plant eaters.

Biologists have discovered that animals which have the same characteristics also eat the same food. If one compares the anatomy of carnivores with our own, it is clearly demonstrated that we were not made to eat meat.

A few typical anatomical characteristics of carnivores, omnivores, plant eaters and humans as a comparison:

Teeth (Incisors)

Meat eaters	Short and pointed
Omnivores	Short and pointed
Plant eaters	Wide, flat, spade-shaped
Humans	Wide, flat, spade-shaped

Stomach acidity

Meat eaters	Less or equal to pH 1 with food in the stomach
Omnivores	Less or equal to pH 1 with food in the stomach
Plant eaters	pH 4-5 with food in the stomach
Humans	pH 4-5 with food in the stomach

Length of the Small Intestine

Meat eaters	3 to 6 times body length
Omnivores	4 to 6 times body length
Plant eaters	10 to more than 12 times body length
Humans	10 to 11 times body length (height)

Dr. Richard Leakey, a well-known anthropologist, summarizes this as follows: "We cannot rip up meat or skin with our hands. Our front teeth were not made to tear meat or skin. We do not have large carnassial teeth (fangs), and we would also not be able to use food sources which require these big fangs."

Source: 8

The Disadvantages of a Diet with Animal Products

Animal products are rich in fat and protein, but provide few carbohydrates and contain **no** fiber.

Thus they make a large contribution toward over-nourishment and being overweight, with all of the negative consequences which result from this; for example, high blood pressure and diabetes.

Animal fats contain a lot of saturated fatty acids, and cholesterol occurs **only** in animal fats.
Saturated fats and cholesterol are to a large extent responsible for the so-called diseases of civilization such as arteriosclerosis.

Note: Cholesterol is important for the human body. But it is not necessary to get it in one's diet, as the body itself is able to produce sufficient amounts of it.

The consequences of arteriosclerosis (heart attacks and strokes) are the number one cause of death in the industrial nations, about 50% of all deaths.
Many people still assume strokes to be an unavoidable fate. They are not aware that up to half of strokes and heart attacks could be avoided by means of preventive measures or by treating the risk factors.

85% of strokes can be attributed to arteriosclerosis, which interferes with circulation.

In a gradual process which takes place over many years, plaque builds up in the blood vessels, including the ones leading to the brain, as well as the others. This plaque narrows the vessels.
A stroke occurs when a blood vessel is completely closed off by a blood clot. The same is true of a heart attack.

Arteriosclerosis is promoted by various factors. These include smoking, lack of exercise, a diet containing too many calories and fats, stress, the immoderate consumption of alcohol, and, in women, the combination of smoking and taking birth control pills.

The consequences of this lifestyle are high blood pressure, abnormally high cholesterol, triglyceride and blood glucose levels, being overweight and diabetes.

Source 9: Swiss Heart Foundation

Preventing Cancer through Diet

… It has long been suspected that nutrition and the development of cancer could be related to each other.
Already at the start of the 20th century doctors were advising their patients to avoid being overweight, and to eat more plant food than animal food, in order to reduce the risk of cancer.

Under contract from the United States Congress, the English scientists Doll and Pet published "The Causes of Cancer" in 1981. Utilizing international epidemiological data concerning the frequency of cancer cases, they came to the conclusion that over 35 percent of all cancer deaths could be blamed on improper nutrition.

This percentage is significantly higher for some types of cancer.
In other words, changing eating habits can aid in the prevention of cancer in general and certain cancers in particular … .

Source 10:   Prof. Dr. h.c. Harald zu Hausen, Chairman and scientific member of the Board of Directors of the Foundation of the German Cancer Research Center, Heidelberg.

Cancer is a preventable disease. Proper nutrition and a healthy lifestyle prevent many common cancers.
A committee of scientists formed by the World Cancer Research Fund (WCRF) and the American Institute for Cancer Research (AICR) has published a 670 page report entitled "Food, Nutrition and the Prevention of Cancer: a global perspective" which utilizes research data from around the world to support the above thesis.

... The influence of diet on the formation of cancers lies primarily in its potential to prevent the occurrence of cancer through the selection of the right foods ...
... Changes in personal diet have, according to current research, a much greater effect on the lowering of the cancer rate than do government measures in the area of food safety, as, for example, regulations regarding the use of additives, comprehensive control of residues and the limitation of certain preparation processes.

The potential of diet in preventing cancer can only be reached when the type and amount of food consumed is changed.
These changes will make their way into the existing social classes, and signify a parting from some habits.

The goal is indeed well defined and the message is clear: More vegetables and fruit, varied meals and a lot of exercise ... .

Source 11: German Institute for Nutritional Research, Potsdam-Rehbrücke (DIFE),
Brochure: Cancer Prevention through Nutrition www.dife.de
(Public foundation and member of the Gottfried Wilhelm Leibniz Scientific Society. The foundation is equally funded by the State of Brandenburg and the German Federal Government.)

Information and studies concerning the positive effects of consuming fruit and vegetables on diseases (as well as their prevention) are appearing ever more frequently:

Researchers have discovered a connection between eating certain plants and lowering the risk of contracting the extremely aggressive pancreatic cancer.

A high level of vegetable consumption lowers the risk of cancer of the pancreas by 50 percent. This was the conclusion of American researchers after a study including more than 2,000 participants. Yellow vegetables as well as those with dark leaves are especially effective against this aggressive cancer.
Eating five small portions of these vegetables is the most effective means of preventing pancreatic cancer.

In their investigation, the researchers asked 2,233 persons, of whom 532 had cancer of the pancreas, how many servings of vegetables or fruit they had eaten during the past year on a daily basis.

The findings: Onions, garlic, beans, yellow vegetables like carrots, corn and sweet potatoes, and also vegetables with dark leaves and cruciferous plants such as cabbage and broccoli did the best job of protecting against pancreatic cancer.

The evaluation of the study revealed that the daily consumption of at least five portions of the protective vegetable and fruit varieties lowered the risk of this type of cancer by 50 percent, when compared with the consumption of a maximum of two portions per day. The scientists found that not only the quantity of these vegetables and fruit consumed was of importance, but also the way in which they were prepared.
Raw vegetables provide better protection than cooked vegetables.

Source: 12

How healthy is meat?

Meat contains antibiotics and hormones. During the digestive process, carcinogenic substances form in the intestines and acid in the metabolization.
Due to the lack of roughage these toxins remain in the intestinal tract longer and thus have more time to do their damage. The consumption of meat is an important risk factor in the development of colon cancer, the second most common kind of cancer.
The consumption of meat leads to an elevated excretion of uric acid in the urine, and thus to a general acidification of the urine, which promotes the formation of kidney stones from uric acid.

Those are only two examples of the role of meat consumption in the development of disease.

The interrelation between the ingestion of red meat/meat products and the occurrence of colon cancer has, in the meantime, been well established.
This effect is especially evident in meat products such as sausage, ham, pickled foods, etc.

Through heating, meat proteins become sources for the formation of carcinogenic heterocyclic amines. In the process of preserving meats by means of pickling and smoking, substances such as N-Nitroso compound are formed, which has mutagenic and toxic effects on genes.

The excessive ingestion of fat is a further risk factor in colon cancer, especially because of the high saturated fat content.

Sources: 13

How healthy are eggs?

Eggs contain practically the highest concentration of cholesterol of any foodstuff. Of course, cholesterol is, as is often gladly pointed out, an important building material for hormones and cell walls. But it is produced by the body itself and, therefore, need not be ingested.

Excess cholesterol is a burden on the body. It interferes with the natural ability of the body to regulate the metabolism of cholesterol.

This plays a role in the constriction of the blood vessels (deposit of plaque -- hardening of the arteries).

Compared with the norm, vegans have a substantially lower level of cholesterol in their blood.

Sources: 13

Cholesterol and Gallstones

In Germany alone it is estimated that there are 5 million people with gallstones. More than twice as many women than men are affected by this.

About 90% of gallstones are cholesterol stones, and are composed of about 70% cholesterol.

The most important risk factors in the formation of gallstones are being overweight, gender and advanced age.

Sources: 13-1

How healthy is milk?

Milk consumption presents innumerable health risks, beginning with direct effects on infants (risk of diabetes) and, later in life, chronic degenerative arterial disease and impairment of the immune system.

Finland has the highest milk and milk product consumption rate and the highest diabetes rate worldwide.

Spain is among the countries of the European Union with the least consumption of milk and milk products and has one of the lowest diabetes rates.

It has been known since the beginning of the nineties that the diabetes rates in a given country increase when milk consumption rises.

Sources: http://www.milchlos.de/milos_0501.htm
medline: Diabetes Care 1991 Nov; 14(11):1081-3 Relationship between cow's milk consumption and incidence of IDDM in childhood. Dahl-Jorgensen K, Joner G, Hanssen KF. Aker Diabetes Research Center, Aker University Hospital, Oslo, Norway.

Cow's milk contains about three times as much protein as mother's milk and almost 50 percent more fat.

No other species still drinks milk after the end of the young offspring phase, and there is no other species which drinks the milk of a different species other than domesticated cats and dogs, which have been made accustomed to this.

Beginning with the fourth year of life most people develop an intolerance for milk, that is, the inability to digest the lactose in the milk; for at this age they can no longer synthesize the digestive enzyme lactase.

Ingesting milk products after the toddler stage can cause diarrhea, flatulence and cramps.

Milk products, such as cheese, milk, butter, cream, yogurt and whey, which one finds in many margarines and commercially baked goods, contribute to the development of heart disease, certain cancers and strokes, because they are rich in fat and cholesterol.

Studies have repeatedly shown that milk products contribute toward osteoporosis.

Source: 14

In addition, milk products attack the important mucous membrane barrier of the intestines, and thus serve to allow unwanted proteins into the organism.

This results in making a person more prone to allergies, some of them quite serious.

Lactose ("milk sugar") Intolerance

Approximately 15 percent of Austrians suffer from unrecognized lactose intolerance. This makes itself increasingly known with age. Usually newborns have a lot of the enzyme lactase. After the end of the nursing stage the concentration of this enzyme diminishes slowly. Most adults have only one tenth of the lactase of infants.

About 70% of Europeans can no longer digest lactose by the age of 60.

Altogether, 75 to 80 percent of the world's population is more or less lactose intolerant.

It is believed that about 12 million people in Germany have some degree of lactose intolerance. It follows that the figure could be as high as 1.2 million people in Austria.

Source 15: Online Magazine Profil.at

What does a "healthy diet" mean?

A healthy diet includes, in addition to taking in the proper number of calories for your needs, choosing foods that are easily digestible, avoiding toxic substances, and, above all, getting all of the vitamins, minerals and trace elements essential to life in sufficient amounts.
Here it is assumed that the individual is aware of the contents of foodstuffs, and in addition, has the readiness and determination to implement this knowledge in his/her daily diet plan.

Just "cooking healthy" on the weekend will probably not meet the body's requirements.
Thus it is important to see that one looks for creative solutions in one's daily life, whether on the job, traveling or meeting other obligations.

A few basic rules for a healthy vegan diet:

1. Eat fruit and vegetables several times per day and in substantial amounts.
   They contain vitamins, minerals, carotene, flavanone, trace elements and fiber. The greatest amount of these is found in fresh fruit and vegetables.

2. You should give preference to whole grain foods.
   Products made with white flour such as cake, crackers and rolls contain almost none of the substances essential to life.

3. Use quality fats and oils.
   Cold-pressed plant oils such as flaxseed oil, hemp oil and walnut oil, which contain the most essential polyunsaturated fatty acids, are among the oils you could choose. No cold-pressed fats should be used for frying foods.

4. Reduce or avoid sugar, alcohol, prepared foods, and canned foods.
   They contain no or few elements necessary to life and can use up minerals in the body.

Fiber explained

Fiber is one of the natural ingredients of foods from plants, while animal foods contain **no** fiber.
The fibers in the plant form a network of frames and supports which give it stability and holding power.
Thus fiber is present in the cell walls and outer tissue of grains, legumes, nuts, fruit and vegetables.

Fiber makes you feel full and causes less of an increase in the blood glucose level, in comparison to low-fiber foodstuffs.
This creates a metabolism which is favorable to weight reduction. Diabetics also profit from it.

One differentiates between soluble and insoluble fiber. Insoluble fiber helps to keep you regular if it is taken with enough liquids. It swells in the intestines and ensures sufficient filling pressure which pushes the chyme along further.

50 grams of insoluble fiber can bind 200-300 grams of water. Therefore it is important to drink enough fluids when you are consuming fibrous foods.

So fiber increases the volume and weight of the contents of the intestines and softens it at the same time.
Fiber stimulates intestinal peristalsis in a natural manner, and ensures the regular emptying of the intestines. But if one does not drink enough liquids, it can have the opposite effect.

To summarize in brief:

Fiber

-- **makes you feel more like you have had enough to eat by filling up the stomach to a greater extent**

-- **delays the emptying of the stomach**

-- **reduces "transit time" in the intestines**

You should eat at least 30 grams of fiber each day

Fiber content of some foods --
(soluble and insoluble combined, in grams per 100 grams)

White rice (cooked)	0.5
Natural rice (cooked)	1.0
Millet, hulled	3.9
Oats, kernels	9.3
Spelt, green kernels	9.9
Rye	13.4
Wheat	9.6
White flour	1.5
Noodles, cooked	1.5
Whole grain noodles, cooked	4.4
Cucumbers	0.9
Tomatoes	1.3
Eggplant	1.4
Onions	1.4
Kohlrabi	1.5
Leek	2.2
Red beets	2.5
Cauliflower	2.9
Carrots	2.9
Broccoli	3.0

LEGUMES –– prepared

Lentils	2.8
Chickpeas	4.4
Green peas	5.0
Navy beans	7.5
Kidney beans	8.3
Banana	2.0
Strawberries	2.0
Orange	2.2
Apple	2.3
Pear	2.8
Walnuts	4.6
Hazelnuts	7.4
Almonds	9.8

Fiber analyses:
German Institute for Grain, Potato and Fat Research, Detmold

Source: 16

Advantages of vegan nutrition and its effects on health

I experience the advantages on different levels:

First advantage:
Feeling well when eating and afterwards.

On this diet, the blood sugar level remains relatively constant; i.e., hunger associated with the consumption of sugar and sleepiness are drastically reduced.

This well-being does not result automatically, as I mentioned, but only because I have made the decision to eat a vegan diet. That means that you have to adhere to the dietary requirements for the supply of vital foodstuff components.

This feeling of well-being is based on several factors which can likely be explained by medical doctors or practitioners of alternative medicine who have the appropriate background (nutrition and sports) -- (see also the chapter on dietary supplements):

-- From where am I starting?
   Do I have to make up for eating an unbalanced diet in the past?
   What foods do I have on hand?
   A detailed blood or hair analysis could yield some clues.
   A blood analysis reflects the diet during the past days and weeks.
   A hair analysis reflects the diet during the past few months.

-- How do my athletic activities affect my need for certain nutrients?
   In determining this, you need to consider the amount of training, body weight and weather conditions (loss of minerals through perspiration).

-- How and with what can I meet my need for nutrients?
   I allow myself to be guided quite consciously by the way my
   body feels in choosing foods. Of course it is nice to know what
   nutrients and how much of them a certain kind of food contains,
   but a table of nutritional values doesn't help me along when I
   want to know when and how much of it I should consume.

-- Is my body capable of absorbing these nutrients?
   Do they ever reach the individual cell?
   If there are well-founded doubts here -- for example, in the
   form of an illness or a chronic dip in performance -- then either
   intensive self study or medical advice will help.

   For example, vitamin B12: There is a lack of it in the
   population as a whole, especially in omnivores, who lack the
   intrinsic factor (enzyme) necessary for its absorption.

Second advantage:
Rapid absorption of the nutritional components.

It is possible to process meals quickly:

-- Fruit and vegetables are generally easy to digest.
   This can result in your feeling hungry after a short while
   (shorter than you are used to). When this happens, I eat a
   snack consisting of fruit or nuts (almonds).

-- At each meal I put the emphasis either on protein or
   carbohydrates.
   Why?

A variety of enzymes, acids, and chemical bases are needed for the digestion of protein and carbohydrates. They are produced by the body.

If you eat both in equal proportion (50:50) and in large amounts, the body produces enzymes to aid in the digestion of both, which causes them to interfere with each other's intended effect.

That is why beans and peas are difficult to digest and can cause flatulence.

But if the proportion of protein and carbohydrates is 75:25 or 80:20 digestion is not interfered with.

-- Limit the varieties of fruit or vegetables to two or three kinds per meal.

Why?

I cannot give any reasons for this.

But my experience has been that a meal sets better with me when I limit the varieties to two or three.

You can test this yourself, and take note of your body's reaction. See if there isn't a difference.

Third advantage:
You will have more energy at your disposal for work or sports.

Fourth advantage:
Health/disease prevention

A carefully planned vegan diet enables the body to bring itself into balance, and so, to heal itself (or to remain healthy).

An example of my diet on a day when I am not training:

Breakfast:
Fruit salad – four bananas, three apples and the juice of two lemons.

Snack:
A large handful of walnuts (sometimes raisins as well).

Lunch:
Lettuce with cucumbers, tomatoes, herbs and lemon juice.
Quinoa (see note below) with tofu, eggplant, onion, carrots.

Snack:
Two bananas and a big handful of almonds.

Dinner:
Rice noodles with tofu, broccoli and onion; the juice of one lemon. (Some days I have bread with soy margarine and cucumbers/ tomatoes).

Note: Quinoa, like amaranth, is described as a gluten-free "pseudo-grain". The protein content (15% -- contains the amino acid cysteine and the essential amino acids lysine and tryptophan) and a few minerals (potassium 710 mg, magnesium 240 mg, iron 10.8 mg per 100 grams) actually exceeds the common kinds of grains.

The fat content (5%) is comprised of 99% polyunsaturated fatty acids, and 50% of that consists of the essential linoleic acid. Grown in Peru and Bolivia.

Sources: 16-1.

What do institutions have to say about diet?

From a considerable amount of epidemiological and clinical data it can be concluded that the liberal consumption of plant foods and complex carbohydrates is associated with a reduction in the risk of diverse chronic ailments.
This concerns primarily coronary heart disease, certain cancers, high blood pressure and diabetes.

Source 17: World Health Organization (WHO)

The American Dietetic Association (ADA) and the Dieticians of Canada (DC) took a stand in 2003 in a joint position paper on the health advantages of vegetarian and vegan nutrition.
The most renowned dietetic scientists of the United States and Canada belong to these organizations.
The ADA alone has about 70,000 members.

To quote from this position paper:

... Well-planned **vegan** and other forms of vegetarian nourishment are suited to all phases of the life cycle, including pregnancy, the lactation period, early and later childhood and adolescence. Vegetarian diets offer a number of advantages ...

... It is the position of the American Dietetic Association (ADA) and the Dieticians of Canada (DC) that a rationally planned vegetarian diet promotes health and is adequate to meet nutritional needs, and is useful for the prevention and treatment of certain diseases ...

... It is the responsibility of nutritional scientists to support and encourage persons who are interested in taking up a vegetarian diet ...

Source 18: ADA Reports   Position of the American Dietetic Association and Dietitians of Canada

The Components of Food

In order to make it easier for you to create a diet it would certainly be helpful to know where and in what amounts food components can be found.

When you are making the change to a vegan diet this will serve to provide support, and help you to "train yourself in" in an area which you may have previously neglected.

Protein

Proteins are the building blocks of the body. They are comprised of various amino acids.

Protein Needs

Nitrogen balance is the decisive factor here. Each day the body builds up and removes proteins.

It takes care of a part of its need for protein through the products of the breakdown process, which it simply splits up into amino acids and uses again. Another part is excreted and must be replaced.

The need for individual essential amino acids varies quite a bit. Age is a factor here. In the infant stage, when the fastest growth is taking place, 2.5 grams (.08 ounces) of essential and non-essential amino acids are needed per kilogram (2.2 pounds) of body weight.

For adults, about one gram (.035 ounces) per kilogram is the estimate, while an athlete requires about 1.5 g/kg (.05 oz) per day.

Power athletes need between 1.6 and 1.8 g (.06 oz) in order to achieve a positive nitrogen balance.

The greater need of an athlete for protein is due partially to muscle growth. In addition, the need for regeneration is increased, this because minor "injuries" occur while the muscles are under stress, and additional protein serves as a building block used in the healing process.

Lastly, amino acids are used as energy in endurance training. These losses also must be made up for.

Which protein is the best?

The quality of the protein sources ingested is of prime importance for the rapidity of muscle growth.

Many people mistakenly believe that meat is the best source of protein.

Our digestive system is of a vegetarian nature. We also have to remember the undesirable by-products of meat consumption that were mentioned.

Taking in "too much" plant protein does not have the negative effects of eating too much meat, because fruit and vegetables do not contain purine and cholesterol.

The variety of amino acids (building blocks of protein) in plant foods is often greater than that of meat.

Soy contains all of the essential amino acids, that is, those that the body cannot produce from other amino acids.

The protein content of some foods --

Soybeans	37-43%	(This is more than meat contains).
Legumes	22-30%	(Also more than meat)
Meat	20-22%	
Grains	7-17%	
Nuts, Seeds	8-17%	
Bread, Potatoes	10%	

Carbohydrates

Carbohydrates carry energy to our bodies. They consist of carbon, oxygen and hydrogen.

Only they can promote the increased production of insulin, one of the most potent of the hormones that are required for muscle growth.
Without insulin the muscles cannot be built up, and the carbohydrates cannot be stored.

All carbohydrates are stored in the body in the form of glycogen, about one third of that in the liver, and the remainder in the muscles.

Altogether somewhat more than one half percent of body weight is stored in the form of carbohydrates.
In a man weighing 80 kg (176 lbs) that would come to 350 or 400 grams (12 or 14 ounces). The brain and nervous system requires 120 grams (4 ounces) of that daily to maintain proper functioning.

There are three types of carbohydrates, and they differ in their effects on the body:

Mono-Saccharides		
Structure	Examples	Where found
Simple Sugar, made up of individual sugar molecules, is available as energy very quickly, but for a very short period of time.	Glucose (blood sugar)	Blood
	Fructose (fruit sugar)	Fruit
	Galactose (a type of milk sugar	Milk products

Oligo-Saccharides		
Structure	Examples	Where found
Consist of two or more sugar molecules, and are broken down at an intermediate rate of speed.	Sucrose (cane sugar)	Cane sugar
	Lactose (milk sugar)	Milk products
	Maltose (malt sugar)	Malt

Poly-Saccharides		
Structure	Examples	Where found
Consist of many sugar molecules, and are broken down over a longer period of time. They provide the body energy on a long-term basis.	Plants: starch, cellulose	Grains
	Milk products	Milk products

Glycemic Index

The Glycemic Index (GI) describes the blood sugar reaction to the ingestion of carbohydrate-containing foodstuffs, and thus, indirectly, the insulin reaction of the body as well.

It tells us how fast the carbohydrates of a given food are absorbed by the body.

The blood sugar-elevating effect of grape sugar serves as a reference value (100). The person being tested is asked to consume enough of a foodstuff so that the 100 gram carbohydrate level is reached.

The GI was already created in the 1980's within the context of diabetes research. It was determined, for example, that white bread causes blood sugar to rise more than plain household sugar. But the difference in blood sugar elevation could not be explained by means of the structure of the carbohydrates (that is, complex or small molecule).

Now the discussion concerning the medical significance of the GI centered on the problem that the GI depended upon numerous factors.
What other foods the foodstuff in question was consumed with played a role, as well as food processing and preparation.
Since then an improvement was made -- the glycemic load was taken into account. This takes into consideration the amount of carbohydrates.

Simple sugar in the blood drives the blood sugar and energy levels up as the person consuming it wishes, but the body tries to compensate for too much of it.

The increased production of insulin then lowers the level of sugar drastically, causing one to feel run-down, tired and hungry.

Only foods with a low Glycemic Index give energy evenly.

Complex carbohydrates have lower GI values than do the more simple carbohydrates. It makes sense to give preference in one's daily diet to foods that have a low or intermediate GI value (recommendations for athletes will be found two paragraphs below).

Assessment of the GI Value

In general, the following calibration is used:

High (normally bad):   GI greater than 70

Medium: between 50 and 70

Low (normally good):   lower than 50

The significance of the GI in heart and circulatory diseases

The relationship between the development of coronary heart disease and the Glycemic Index or Glycemic Load was discovered in a large study done in the United States. It is suspected that elevated blood sugar values after eating create "oxidative stress" (see the chapter on food supplements for an explanation) which damages the blood vessels.

It was further noted that the GI also plays a role in lipid levels and for the inflammation marker. After several weeks of eating foods with a low GI the majority of the studies found reduced levels of triglycerides and LDL cholesterol.

The significance of the GI for athletes

The GI is becoming increasingly more important for athletes. Depending upon whether I am in a training or competition stage, I must consume different carbohydrates.

In the daily diet

In so far as possible, foods with a low or medium GI. A high GI leads to faster storage of glycogen, but burdens the body through the higher secretion of insulin, and soon causes one to feel hungry.

After training

Prefer foods with a high or medium GI, in order to replenish the carbohydrate reserves as quickly as possible.

In competition

Primarily foods with a high GI, in order to ensure rapid readying of energy for use (millet, dried fruit, very ripe bananas, malt dextrin).

> When energy bars or drinks were ingested before competition, it resulted in the glucose level falling before the event, and in the emptying of the glycogen stores as well as a rapid reduction of free fatty acids. This was established by studies, which also showed that this condition led to the athlete becoming fatigued sooner.

The Glycemic Index of some foods

It should be noted that the GI can vary according to the manner in which the food is prepared.

High: GI greater than 70	
Sugar from grapes 100	Savory biscuits 85
Dried dates 99	Pretzels 85
French fries, potato starch 95	Ketchup 80
Malt dextrin 95	White flour (baguette) 75
Baked potatoes 95	Pumpkin 75
Sweetened fruit juices 90	Millet 71

Medium: GI between 50 and 70	
Chocolate bar 70	Red beets 64
Noodles and ravioli 70	Pastries, muffins 62
Pineapple 66	Ice cream 61
Orange juice concentrate 65	Long grain rice 60
Bread made from more than one kind of flour, barley bread 65	Buckwheat, unripe spelt grain 55
Bananas, raisins 65	Brown rice, basmati rice 50

Low: GI lower than 50	
Grapefruit juice 48	Amaranth 30
Chickpeas (canned) 41	Dried peas 22
Kidney beans 40	Nuts, almonds 22
Peas, fresh 40	Soy bean sprouts, cooked 20
Fruit juices, freshly pressed (without sugar) 40	Lemons 15
Green mung beans 38	Avocado 20
Dates/Figs, fresh 40	Mushrooms, asparagus 15
Quinoa, rye 35	Vegetable juice, fresh 15
Oranges, pears 35	Onions, garlic 10
Horseradish 35	Tomatoes, peppers 10
Chickpeas 30	Cabbage, leeks, broccoli 10
Green beans, fresh 30	Fresh vegetables, lettuce 10
Apple, peach, fresh fruit, nectarine 30	Eggplant, zucchini 10

A statistical analysis points toward a relationship between a high blood sugar level and an increased risk of cancer.

Over 1.3 million persons between the ages of 30 and 95 were observed in a long-term Korean study.

The scientists evaluated the data of government employees and their dependents.
Blood samples were taken regularly and their smoking and alcohol consumption were recorded on questionnaires.

Over a period of ten years the researchers kept track of the number of cancer cases, comparing the study participants having a blood glucose level of over 140 mg per deciliter with those who were under 90 mg.

The risk of cancer in those with a high blood sugar level was 29% higher than the control group in men; and, in women, 23% higher.

Approximately 150 million people suffer from diabetes world-wide.

Scientists say that this figure could double by the year 2025. While there is conclusive evidence that there is a connection between diabetes and an increased risk of heart and circulatory diseases, this has not yet been established in the case of diabetes and cancer.

Source: 19

Fats

Fat is a chemical compound made up of various fatty acids, fats and oils which are obtained from plant or animal cells or produced synthetically.
Fats are among the basic nutritive materials in the diet.

A total of 68% of the population of the industrial nations dies of fat-intake related illnesses, including heart and circulatory diseases (43.8%), cancer (22.4%) and diabetes (1.8%). About 50% of this population is overweight.

But during the past few years it has been determined that carbohydrates can be implicated at least as much as fat in the development of morbid obesity, and that, above all, the consumption of carbohydrates in combination with fat is very hazardous to health.
www.channing.harvard.edu/nhs/history/index.shtml#histI
(Nurses' Health Study)
The amount and type of fat consumed, just as is the case with carbohydrates, determines whether we become healthy, energetic, strong and slender, or if the opposite turns out to be the case.

Fat is primarily a provider of energy. But because we hardly use up any fat energy in today's lifestyle and sedentary occupations, we store the fat in the body like a cushion.
Yet we cannot refrain from eating fat, for it is (as are proteins) a component of cell membranes, almost all body cells, and, most importantly, the main component of nerve and brain cells.
In addition, fat is essential for the formation of hormones, the ability of the blood to flow, the protection of internal organs and numerous important body functions.

High quality fatty acids are very important for health, growth, performance -- yes, indispensable for life in general.
But we need the right amount of fat (too little is just as damaging as too much) and, above all, we need the proper fats.

Different fatty acids and their effects

Fat consists of various fatty acids and these determine whether:

-- a fat is healthy,

-- it is primarily a provider of energy,

-- whether it is stored as body fat or not,

-- if it is used more for the formation of hormones,

-- or if it is used more for the healthy development of the brain,

-- it serves to promote the optimal growth of the body.

In principle, only linoleic acid (an Omega-6 fatty acid) and Alpha linolenic acid (an Omega-3 fatty acid) are essential, which means that they must be ingested.
The body can produce itself or synthesize all other fatty acids necessary for maintaining good health from these two fatty acids.

Even the often criticized "saturated" fatty acids, which we get in our food, optimize metabolism, although it is true that they are not necessary for life.
The fact that optimal growth takes place when 30% saturated and 70% polyunsaturated fats are taken in speaks for the notion that there is also a need for non-essential saturated fatty acids.

The dangerous fat-carbohydrate combination

Carbohydrates, especially refined carbohydrates; that is, sugars and syrups, but also refined starch like white rice, white flour, white bread, rice cakes and sweetened fruit juices -- all of them carbohydrate products with a high Glycemic Index (GI) -- can be very easily converted by the organism into fat with saturated fatty acids (palmitic acid) and cholesterol.

Thus, if you take in too many of these carbohydrates, you automatically upset the natural fatty acid balance and just as automatically raise the amount of fat in the body above the amount of ingested pure fatty acids.

Meanwhile there is more and more evidence that excess weight is only 10% a problem of genuine overeating, but 90% of it can be traced back to the lack of certain nutrients (above all, Omega-3 fatty acids, chromium, iodine, potassium, magnesium, calcium and fiber).

These deficiencies lead to hunger or even ravenous hunger, which then leads to excessive eating.
They slow down metabolism, so that fewer calories are consumed and, in the end, the result is being overweight.

Fat in endurance sports

Athletes often make the mistake of eating a low-fat diet, this because they believe that in this way they will build up more muscle and less body fat.
When it comes to sports, fatty acids perform the following tasks: They produce energy in all of the body's cells, which in turn is important for performance capacity, the building of muscle and regeneration from training.

No one burns up as much fat as an endurance athlete, whether he/she is resting or training.

During serious preparatory training (fat metabolism training) 40-50% of fat is burned off.

If only 25% of one's diet consists of fat, it will inevitably lead to an imbalance between fat intake and fat usage, and thus in the long run to a reduction in fat stored in the body.
This fact, which, on the surface, appears to be desirable, has a big disadvantage: In these circumstances the danger of a negative energy balance developing is great, for there is no naturally felt need to take in carbohydrates and protein in the excessive amounts which are then required.

As the sources of different cell hormones, fatty acids play an important role in the regulation of clotting and inflammatory processes, as well as in the opening up and constriction of blood vessels.

Fatty acids are incorporated into the cell membranes in approximately the same proportion in which they are found in the fats of foodstuff. The type of fatty acids found there directly influences the functions of cell membranes (material exchange, shaping, enzyme activities).

An unfavorable combination of the fats from foods, as is typical for a "normal" diet, can significantly impair the cell's ability to carry out these functions.

As the exchange of fats in the cell wall transpires relatively slowly, one must stay with a change in the fatty acid composition of the food consumed for a long time and on a regular basis, if one wishes to achieve a favorable change in these functions!

Improving the quality of fat intake

Depending upon food composition, fats can promote either processes that cause illness or ones that protect.

The consequences of "normal" nourishment:
Processes which lead to illness are aided by the excessive intake of animal fats, which contain a high proportion of saturated fatty acids, cholesterol, purines (promote the formation of uric acid) and arachidonic acid (plays an important role in the development of heart disease, arthritis and immune deficiencies).

The same is true of foods which are rich in so-called trans fatty acids. These are formed naturally in small amounts in, for example, milk and butter; and in large amounts in the artificial production of hydrogenated fats (fats for frying and baking, margarine). Today they are uniformly considered to be undesirable if one wants to have good health.

Next to hazelnut oil, olive oil has the highest proportion of Oleic acid of all foodstuffs. It is the ideal fat for both warm and cold meals, and should replace hydrogenated fats. It is easily digestible and ideally suited to the preparation of salads.
The easy digestibility of Mediterranean meals has been known for a long time, as well as the fact that heart and circulatory diseases are less common in these countries than, for example, in central or eastern European countries.

Two factors are responsible for this: More vegetables and fruit are eaten by the Mediterranean peoples, and the high proportion of fat from oil in their total fat intake.

The Omega-3 fatty acids, which are among the polyunsaturated fatty acids, have been proven to inhibit the emergence and progress of various disease processes, such as heart disease, inflammation processes and immune deficiencies.

Unfortunately, the intake of Omega-3 fatty acids is highly insufficient in the normal diet.

The proportion of Omega-6 to Omega-3 fatty acids is usually more than 10:1, but should be less than 5:1.
Because only a few foods have a high Omega-3 fatty acid content (in other words, a ratio of less than 5:1), these fatty acids should definitely be integrated into the daily menu in larger amounts.

Essential fatty acids
(These must be present in the diet)

Omega-3 fatty acids

-- Linolenic acid
   found in linseed oil, flax oil, hemp oil

Omega-6 fatty acids

-- Linoleic acid
   found in linseed oil, flax oil, sunflower oil

If the body is provided with di-unsaturated fatty acids, it is able to produce tri-unsaturated fats, which are important for life.

Good, valuable cooking oils must be cold-pressed, as only in this manner can the important polyunsaturated fatty acids be retained, as well as the vitamins, which are easily ruined.

The Fatty Acid Content of a Few Kinds of Oil

	Satu-rated Fatty Acids	Mono-Unsat-urated Fatty Acids	Di-Unsat-urated Fatty Acids	Tri-Unsat-urated Fatty Acids	
		Oleic Acid	Linoleic Acid	Gamma Linolenic Acid	Alpha Linolenic Acid
		OMEGA 9	OMEGA 6	OMEGA 6	OMEGA 3
Thistle oil	10%	13%	76%	1%	-
Hemp oil	-	-	50-70%	2-4%	15-25%
Hazelnut oil	8%	78%	14%	-	-
Pumpkin seed oil	19%	28%	53%	-	-
Flax oil	10%	17%	15%	-	58%
Olive oil	15%	76%	9%	-	-
Rapeseed oil	6%	69%	20%	-	9%
Sunflower oil	10%	30%	60%	-	-
Walnut oil	6%	24%	55%	6%	9%

Source: 20

Most health food stores are well-stocked with oils.

Highly nutritious oils are also automatically absorbed through the consumption of the corresponding foods (nuts, for example).

The nutritional value of nuts

In recent years several epidemiological studies have shown a reduced risk of heart and circulatory diseases when the ingestion of nuts is increased.

Clinical studies indicate that this effect is based either partially or completely on the lowering of the total cholesterol and LDL cholesterol levels in the blood as a result of consuming nuts.
It is still not clear what it is about nuts that has this effect, but much of the evidence points to the favorable fatty acid profile of nuts (relatively high content of mono-unsaturated and poly-unsaturated fatty acids).

These investigations have primarily been carried out in the United States, and there they have brought about a significant change in the evaluation of nut consumption by nutritional scientists and consultants.

The previous more negative view ("calorie bombs") has given way to the explicit approval of increased nut consumption.

Europeans, for the most part, have not taken note of this change.

There has been only one European epidemiological study concerning the influence of nut consumption on risk factors for heart and circulatory diseases, this by scientists at Grenoble University (Lavedrine et al., 1999).
In the Dauphiné area walnut production plays a significant role in the economy, walnut consumption is relatively high and walnut oil is used a lot in the preparation of salads.

Here, the lipid levels in about 800 men and women aged 18-65 were determined, and the consumption of walnuts and walnut oil was investigated.

In persons who frequently consumed these foodstuffs, HDL cholesterol and apolipoprotein A-1 (apoA1) levels were clearly higher than in those with limited consumption.

A protective effect against heart and circulatory diseases is attributed to these substances (Mensink and Katan, 1989; Dreon *et al.*, 1990; Kris-Etherton *et al.*, 1999).

This effect was directly related to the quantity of walnut and walnut oil intake.

The findings of some epidemiological studies also indicate a positive influence of nut consumption on cancer risk.

The evaluation of cancer and diet statistics in 59 countries over a time span of 5 years, 1985-89, showed that the more nuts and oil seeds were consumed, the lower the morbidity rate from prostate cancer dropped (Hebert *et al.*, 1998).

For over 20 years about 120,000 American nurses participated in the Nurses' Health Study, providing information concerning their lifestyle and health status. After the exclusion of those who returned their questionnaires without having filled them out completely or who were already suffering from various serious diseases at the start of the study, approximately 86,000 women between the ages of 34 and 59 remained. These were further observed.

During a time span of 14 years there were 861 non-fatal and 394 fatal heart attacks among these participants. The results of other epidemiological studies regarding the relationship between the consumption of nuts were confirmed. When nuts were consumed frequently (140 grams per week or more) the relative risk of fatal heart attacks was reduced by 39%, and that of non-fatal heart attacks by 32% (Hu *et al.*, 1998).

Source 21: Federal Research Institute for Nutrition, Karlsruhe

Walnuts

Walnuts are different from other varieties of nuts in that they contain a larger amount of polyunsaturated fatty acids, among others, alpha-linolenic acid, which belongs to the Omega-3 fatty acids, which the human organism needs.

In addition, walnuts contain many substances that promote good health, such as vitamin E, folic acid, plant fiber, polyphenols (which are counted among the so-called secondary plant nutrients; see above) and other tannins.

Along with the favorable fatty acid profile, it is also the great amount of arginine, an amino acid, that makes walnuts one of the most valuable foods for the brain.

50 grams or 1.75 ounces of walnuts are sufficient to meet the daily requirement of Omega-3 fatty acids for an adult.

Fatty acid profile of walnuts

100 g walnuts contain 68 g fat of that:
saturated fatty acids	7.1 g
mono-unsaturated fatty acids	10 g
polyunsaturated fatty acids	50 g

Fatty acid profile of almonds

Almonds contain a lot of vitamin B and vitamin E. They have the highest amount of the following minerals of all nuts: calcium (252 mg), magnesium (170 mg) and potassium (835 mg).

100 grams of almonds contain 58 g fat of that:
saturated fatty acids	2.9 g
mono-unsaturated fatty acids	46.4 g
polyunsaturated fatty acids	8.7 g

Vitamins
(the most important)

Vitamin A   (retinol)
Important for: eyes, skin, mucous membranes.
Found in: spinach, broccoli, kale.
(the body produces vitamin A from beta-carotene)

Vitamin B1   (thiamin)
Important for: nerves, carbohydrate metabolism.
Found in: wheat germ, whole grain bread, potatoes, legumes.

Vitamin B2   (riboflavin or lactoflavin)
Important for: skin and mucous membranes, metabolism of fats,
carbohydrates and proteins.
Found in: whole grain products, broccoli, asparagus, spinach.

Vitamin B3   (niacin)
Important for: metabolism of carbohydrates and fats.
Found in: whole grain products.

Vitamin B5   (pantothenic acid)
Important for: fat, carbohydrate and protein metabolism.
Found in: broccoli, cauliflower, whole grain products, nuts.

Vitamin B6   (pyridoxine)
Important for: nervous system, protein metabolism.
Found in: whole grain products, lentils, beans, nuts, bananas.

Vitamin B7   (biotin or Vitamin H)
Important for: skin, hair, nails.
Found in: soy beans, wheat germ.

Vitamin B9   (folic acid)
Important for:
cell regeneration, formation of white and red blood cells.
Found in: whole grain products, greens, tomatoes, soy beans,
nuts, little in fruit.

Vitamin B12 (cobalimin)
Important for: formation of red blood cells.
Found in: This vitamin is only produced by bacteria which live in
the ground or in human or animal intestines.
In the small intestine of some people B12 producing bacteria are
found. At least theoretically, the vitamin can be absorbed from
there.
It remains to be determined what contribution this makes to the
daily intake of vitamin B12 of vegans. Presently, enriched foods
are considered to be the most dependable sources of B12 for
vegans.
Or from preparations: Cynacobalamin is vegan. Hydroxocobalamin
is usually a liver extract, and thus not vegan.

Vitamin C   (ascorbic acid)
Important for: immune system, connective tissue.
Found in: mostly in fresh fruit and vegetables -- for example,
citrus fruits, currants, peppers, green tea, kale.

Vitamin D   (calciferol)
Important for: formation of bone, teeth.
Found in:
ultra-violet light from the sun -- 15 minutes per day suffice.

Vitamin E   (tocopherol)
Important for: cell protection, disease prevention.
Found in: plant oils, nuts, peas, grains, kale.

Vitamin K   (phylochinon)
Important for: lotting of the blood, bone formation.
Found in: green-leaf vegetables, lettuce, tomatoes, cauliflower.

Minerals and Trace Elements

Illness as a result of a lack of minerals?!
It seems rather paradoxical that people in the industrialized nations should suffer from a lack of nutrients.

Yet, this deficiency provides fertile ground for the so-called diseases of civilization such as diabetes, arthritis, heart attacks and cancer. There are widely found hidden deficiencies which do not cause any specific complaints.

Today it is known that a lack of minerals like calcium, magnesium, zinc and selenium helps to cause heart attacks and strokes, and that a chronic shortage of calcium causes osteoporosis and arteriosclerosis.

However, a lack of minerals is seldom the main cause of such serious diseases.
Usually there are additional factors, such as a negative attitude to life, one's physical constitution, lifestyle, as well as the individual's environment and a one-sided diet of unnatural or processed foods.

Calcium

99% of it is found in the bones and teeth. 1% is an important factor in numerous processes such as metabolism, bone mineralization, maintenance of water and electrolyte balance, muscle contraction, the reactions and functioning of nerves and enzymes, as well as clotting of the blood.
Magnesium plays an important role in the level of calcium. Proper magnesium intake supports the absorption of calcium.

Taking in too much magnesium is useless. In fact, it reduces the absorption of calcium.

When it is prepared with calcium sulphate, tofu contains more than four times as much calcium than does cow's milk (be sure to check the label).

There is a lot of calcium in:

tofu, vegetables with green leaves, kale, sesame seeds and tahine.

Calcium content in mg per 100 g of some foods --

Sesame seeds	1500
Soy beans	257
Parsley	245
Kale	230
Nuts	225-234
Figs, dried	160
Cow's milk	120
Broccoli	113

Chromium

There are indications that low chromium intake could be responsible for disturbances in glucose tolerance and for an elevated insulin level in persons with mild hyperglycemia, and that increasing chromium intake could prevent type II diabetes.

The most chromium is contained in:
whole grain products, beans, brewer's yeast and nuts.

Iron

Iron is a component of hemoglobin and myoglobin, two protein molecules whose important biological role is the transport of oxygen and carbon dioxide in the blood.

Only about 10% of the iron present in food is absorbed.

In addition, various food ingredients, when combined with iron, create compounds that are not readily soluble, and thus lower the absorption rate.

Among these are:
Phytin: grains, rice, soy flour.
Oxalate: spinach, rhubarb, alginate from pudding powder,
            instant soups, tannin from black tea, antibiotics,
            antacids (medications that neutralize stomach acid).

The absorption of iron can also be reduced by the excessive ingestion of vitamin B1, a lack of B6, and the constant consumption of large amounts of phosphorous, zinc, copper and manganese.

For the support of iron processing:
-- Vinegar and lemon
   acid aids in the absorption of iron
-- Vitamin C
   taken with iron-rich foodstuffs, it can raise the amount of iron
   absorbed by a factor of 10
-- Foods containing much protein

Foods with high iron content:
quinoa 10.8 g, millet 9 mg, amaranth 9 mg / 100 g, chives, sesame seeds, legumes, nuts, whole grain products, wheat germ, vegetables with green leaves, dried fruit, whole grains, seeds.
To compare: wheat 4.5 mg, rice 3.3 mg, corn 1.9 mg / 100 g.

Using iron pots and pans also contributes to iron intake.
An iron deficiency in the diet is partially compensated for by increased absorption.

Iodine

Fruit and vegetables contain hardly any iodine at all. The most reliable suppliers of iodine are ocean algae like nori, kelp, wakame, and hiziki. All of these are rich in iodine.

Pay attention to the dosage:
-- Nori contains 5-8 mg of iodine per 100 g.
-- Wakame 10 mg

You should take into account foods that contain iodine (bread, salt, prepared foods) and your personal constitution when taking iodine, for there is a certain danger of thyroid gland malfunction.
If you are in doubt, you should seek advice from a doctor.

Potassium

Together with sodium, potassium guides the body's "electricity". Thus, many of the problems which are brought about by a lack of potassium cause symptoms such as muscle weakness. Paralysis can also result.
Tiredness and exhaustion, headaches, weak circulation and low blood pressure, elevated cholesterol levels, kidney impairment, edema (water collecting in the tissue) are further possible complaints.
Plant foods generally have a higher proportion of potassium to sodium.
There is substantial agreement that the evidence points toward an increase in potassium intake being accompanied by a lowering of blood pressure and the reduced probability of a stroke.

Potassium content in mg per 100 g of some foods --

Soy beans	1740
Cocoa powder	1500
Navy beans	1310
Parsley	1000
Nuts	450-740
Bananas	382

Sodium

People eating a "normal" diet are getting about ten times more sodium than they actually need.
8-10 grams of cooking salt absorb about one liter of water in the body, and, in this way, raise the volume of blood, thus causing the blood pressure to rise.

Sodium-rich and potassium-poor diets are dehydrating. You only lose water weight -- there is no reduction in fat.

Potassium is the opponent of sodium, and ensures that more water is eliminated. A poor potassium-sodium balance causes fatigue.

In a "normal" diet, 80% of the salt absorbed daily is hidden in highly processed foods.

Ratio	Potassium	:	Sodium
Bananas	440		1
Oranges	260		1
Watermelon	160		1
Potatoes	110		1
Apples	90		1
Fish	3		1
Meat	3		1
Milk	3		1
Bread	1		3
Salami	1		4
Ham	1		5
Camembert cheese	1		9
Pretzel sticks	1		20

Cobalt

We can only get cobalt in the form of vitamin B12.

Copper

Contained in: bread and other grain products, vegetables, wheat germ, nuts, seeds.

Magnesium

After potassium, magnesium is the second most important intra-cellular (found in the cells) mineral.
Potassium and magnesium from fruit and vegetables can normalize blood pressure in 75% of people with high blood pressure.

Found in 300 enzymes, magnesium is permanently involved in thousands of metabolic reactions.
Magnesium helps alleviate stress -- it is the salt of inner peace.
The more one has of it, the better the internal "power plants" operate -- the mitochondria.
Fatigue and lag in performance disappear.

A lack of magnesium can be due to dietary errors or the increased need for it; for example, when one is under stress or engaged in sports.

Magnesium content of some foods in mg per 100 g --

Wheat bran	590
Cocoa powder	500
Flaxseed	380
Wheat germ	308
Almonds	252
Soy beans	247
Millet	170

The most magnesium is found in nuts, whole grains, oats, millet, brown rice, wheat germ and soy flour.

Manganese

Plant foods are substantially better sources than animal products.
Good sources of manganese are:
nuts, whole grain products, spices, tea.

Phosphorous

Phosphorous is needed in all cells for the tapping of the energy they hold.
Contained in: nuts, whole grains.

Selenium

Scientists believe selenium to be the best partner for vitamin E. It promotes the transport of this vitamin to the cells, and thus prevents gene damage. This trace element aids in the removal of harmful compounds from our bodies. It protects against the effects of toxic substances such as lead, cadmium and mercury.
This is achieved through drawing them out of the connective tissue. Anti-oxidants such as vitamins C and E are also needed at the same time to help eliminate these substances from the body.

A lack of selenium leads to weakness of the immune system. This trace element is of great significance in combating cancer and heart attacks.
Sources of selenium: yeast, garlic, legumes, natural rice, Brazil nuts, nuts, seeds, soy beans, mushrooms, grains, bananas.
High sulfur intake, lack of vitamin E and vitamin B6 bring about a shortage of selenium.

Zinc

The body lays in only a minimum reserve. Zinc helps to render toxins harmless, and is involved in the production of defense substances and defense cells like lymphocytes. About 160 enzymes require zinc. It is directly involved in the building up of protein for new cells -- wounds after operations or injuries heal more quickly.
Excessive amounts of calcium, phosphorous or copper impede the absorption of zinc.

Smokers and even passive smokers often have too little zinc. The excessive consumption of alcohol, stress, sleep disturbances and working the "graveyard shift" have the same effect.

Foods rich in zinc:
wheat germ, lentils, rolled oats, peas, cocoa, whole grain bread.

The Mineral Content of Foodstuffs

Minerals in the ground

Plants take nutrients and minerals out of the ground. In harvesting, the nutrients are in fact carried out of the field. Depending upon the amount of nutrients in the soil it is exhausted after just a few harvests, if it is not fertilized. And the deciding question is found precisely here: Is only nitrogen used, to make the plants grow nice and big, or also the other minerals that we humans require?

From the official side -- German Association for Nutrition (DGE) -- a study was conducted, in which it was determined that exhausted fields are not to be found in Germany (of course, the DGE is commonly known to be an institution sponsored by the food industry).

Only 8 plant foods were investigated in the study.

Source: 22

Obstacles in obtaining sufficient minerals

Environmental pollutants, harmful substances, and pesticides in the air and/or in foodstuffs frequently block the metabolic absorption of minerals.

For example, magnesium does not make it into the blood through the intestinal wall, but rather, is excreted, when there are even small disturbances in the digestive tract (mild inflammation, smoking, alcohol).

Mineral and vitamin content of foods

The nutritional content of foods is, to a large extent, dependent on soil, climate, variety and the time of harvesting.
While the food is being transported, (sometimes several thousand miles), minerals and vitamins are lost. This is also due to further processing, preservatives, etc.
In fruit preserves, for example, 20-25% of the calcium is lost.

Storage and the kind of preparation are important factors which one can influence oneself:
light, oxygen, water and heat destroy nutrients.

Estimated loss of vitamin C:
storing greens in the basement at 12 degrees Celsius (= 53 degrees Fahrenheit), 1 day   40%
storing greens in the refrigerator at 4 degrees (= 39 degrees Fahrenheit),   1 day   25%

loss as a result of washing in running water and slicing 35%,
rinsing in standing water, unsliced, 5 minutes   0.5%

cooking in water with salt at 100 degrees Celsius   55%,
steaming at 100 degrees (212 degrees Fahrenheit – the boiling point)   17%

Recommendation:
-- Buy fresh vegetables shortly before using them
-- Keep in the refrigerator at 4 degrees Celsius only for a
   short time
-- Simmer the vegetables but do not overcook (they should
   remain firm)
-- Or, use a wok: quickly and at a high temperature

Source 23: Swiss Association for Nutrition

Should Dietary Supplements Be Used?

I am of the confirmed opinion that vitamins, minerals and trace elements should be obtained from food.

The vital nutrients contained in fruit, vegetables, grains, etc. are present in the dosages and composition that the body has learned to handle and can process (viewed from the standpoint of evolutionary history).

Using supplements puts the body in a new situation. High doses of isolated nutrients are taken in for a long period of time.

Several studies have revealed that artificially ingested anti-oxidants can upset the balance of oxidants, for the anti-oxidants are present in excess.

In these studies, this led to increased illness and morbidity rates.

Source 24: Studies of Antioxidants

The biochemical processes in the body are much more complexly structured than was previously thought.

For example, taking calcium supplements aids in the uptake of copper, but reduces the absorption of zinc.

It is not possible for us to find the correct balance, due to the great variety of interactions of individual nutrients with the existing enzymes occurring naturally in the body.

The body merely makes the best of the situation and regulates all processes as well as it can.

But it cannot make up for the effects of an unhealthy lifestyle or dietary mistakes.

In my opinion, the goal should be to ensure the provision of vital nutrients with a healthy and many-sided vegan diet. You should only resort to using supplements for a short period of time, and this only when an increased need is present; for example, before a competition or when you are ill.

The question of whether or not to use dietary supplements cannot be answered with a simple "Yes" or "No". It depends on your personal situation (sports, homelife, profession, health).
At times it is not only important to take supplements but also absolutely necessary.

Studies by the producers of dietary supplements should be questioned critically, because a producer has a financial interest in selling his products.
Therefore, a healthy skepticism regarding statements made in advertising is called for.

What procedure should I follow if I choose to supplement my diet?

The basis for a decision to use supplements could/should be a precise analysis of your situation or preliminary testing of individual vitamins and/or minerals.

Should I self-medicate or seek professional advice?

Self-medication

Multi-vitamin preparations

Taking these products is supposed to take care of all possible deficiencies in one fell swoop.

But there are differences among the products made by different manufacturers as regards ingredients, the concentration of vitamins or minerals and the ability of the body to absorb them.

Disadvantage: Your personal situation is not taken into account here.

Mono-preparations

These are isolated minerals such as calcium (for example, as calcium citrate -- note: a citrate is a salt of citric acid).

Often it can be determined where a certain deficit exists by taking individual minerals or vitamins. You could, for example, keep on training the same way and take calcium, observing its effect.

The advantage of mono-preparations lies in the fact that you normally are not ingesting sweeteners, food coloring, etc.

In addition, you learn to better perceive the needs of your own body. What, for example, do I need after a competition, what physical change takes place, does my reaction provide a clue about what I should be eating, do I need more foods that contain a certain mineral ... ?

I recommend a three month trial period. In the case of serious deficiencies this can be too short, as the body needs 1-3 months to refill its stores.

After that, it can make sense to take the preparation for three more months, so that the damage to the organs can be repaired and the body can experience a revitalization.

Important Note:

You should reevaluate after having taken a supplement for a long period of time, for an excess can not only be a burden for the body, but can also cause other deficits.

Supplementing without taking your personal situation into account can be very hazardous to your health.

An example: Many preparations contain a high dosage of calcium in order to prevent osteoporosis. But calcium lowers the level of magnesium, and, as its opponent, interferes with the action of magnesium.

To put it concretely: Taking calcium can cause the problem it is supposed to prevent -- osteoporosis -- this by upsetting the balance between the two minerals.

You should also pay attention to other mineral ratios.

Source 25: Zeitschrift CO'MED

Professional Support

Here, having your personal nutritional needs analyzed is the focus. The second question, which may be even more important, can only be answered by an expert:

Is the absorption of the vital nutrients in the required amount possible in your personal situation, and are these substances being delivered to the places where they are needed (muscle cells, organs, ...)?

Examples of dietary tests:

Blood test

This will reveal what nutrients have entered your blood during recent days/weeks.

The disadvantage of this testing method:

The amount of nutrients in the blood says nothing about the supply of them to the cells, which is all-important for the optimal functioning and performance capacity of, for example, muscles or bones.

The quality of the analysis of the test results is dependent on the experience and specific background of the individual who is advising the athlete. Is he/she personally involved in performance sports?

Mineral analysis of the hair

This will yield data concerning mineral intake over the last several months.
Advantage: Covers a longer time period, heavy metal concentrations are recorded and mineral absorption by the cells is investigated.
There are differences in the spectrum covered among the providers of such laboratory analyses:

-- one provider determines the values for 23 minerals, 15 heavy metals and calculates 5 ratios.

-- another provider determines the values for 30 minerals, 8 toxic mineral substances (heavy metals) and calculates 16 ratios.

One of the ratios is that of iron to copper. Low amounts of copper, manganese and chromium indicate difficulties in the processing of fats. This is the result of an endocrine imbalance.

A low level of magnesium compared to calcium can lead to crystallization of calcium (osteoporosis), and to the depositing of calcium in the urinary tract and gall bladder (kidney and gall stones).

Hair analysis normally is much more informative than a blood test, because a longer period of time is covered and more minerals are tested for.

Boron, for example, is not checked for in a blood analysis, unless there is a concrete reason to do this.
But a lack of boron leads to a loss of calcium and magnesium via the urine. Calcium and magnesium are important elements which are involved in muscular response. Thus, it is also important for an athlete to have a sufficient supply of boron.

The disadvantage of this testing method:

The supply of vitamins is not tested. Whether and why the absorption of nutrients or the transport of vital substances has been disrupted is also not analyzed.

Nano-particle – blood analysis

With this method, the vital nutrient content (vitamins, minerals) is analyzed. In addition, nano-particles in the blood are detected and described by means of specialized microscopic processes as well as radiological tests (analysis of metabolic processes on the cellular level -- structuring and interaction).

This makes it possible to state whether there is sufficient provision of vital substances (especially important for athletes, who have an increased need for these nutrients). This is accomplished by the analysis of metabolic products, which are related to the individual's basal metabolism.

Specifically, the following are tested for:

-- Are sufficient amounts of vital substances being made available to the body?

-- Can enough essential nutrients be absorbed through the digestive tract?

-- Are these substances reaching the places where they are needed?

-- Are our cells able to use them properly?

Using these findings, deficiencies can be precisely balanced out, and their creation can be prevented therapeutically.

The disadvantage of this testing method:
The supply of minerals is not tested over a long time period, and the mineral ratios are not analyzed.

Free radical test

Free radicals are being mentioned ever more frequently in relation to the origin of various diseases, arteriosclerosis and cancer in particular.
Free radicals are aggressive, harmful substances that damage healthy cells, and can destroy them. Thus they bear part of the responsibility for the development and progression of numerous diseases.
The test reveals the occurrence of free radicals, and in this manner whether sufficient vital substances are available to the body.

The disadvantage of this testing method:
The test does not show the cause of the current situation -- whether too few vital nutrients are being absorbed, whether they are being used up at work, in sports, etc, or whether or why the absorption of nutrients or the transportation of vital substances are being disrupted.

Explanation of oxidative stress:

Because reactive oxygen compounds also are created in normal metabolic processes, the development of protective mechanisms was necessary in human evolution.
Normally there is a balance between oxidative and reductive processes.
But if the oxidative reactions are predominant, one speaks of "oxidative stress".

The following factors, among others, cause oxidative stress:

Nicotine, alcohol, ionizing radiation (television, computer monitor, cell phone, ultra-violet rays), ozone, smog, one-sided diets (too few vitamins) with a lot of animal fats.

Anti-oxidants "catch" free radicals and render them harmless. They are found in citrus fruits and many kinds of vegetables (tomatoes, whole-grain rice, nuts, broccoli, ...).
Omega-3 fatty acids also make free radicals harmless. They are found in linseed oil, hemp oil, walnuts, walnut oil and other foodstuffs as well.

Bone density measurement

There are different methods of measurement -- the DXA and DPA evaluations of the hip bones and the spine are very precise. Ultra-sound is too imprecise.
Bone density can also be determined by analyzing the urine.

The result provides information concerning excessive acid content in the body, the danger of osteoporosis and the supply of calcium and vitamin D.

The disadvantage of this method of testing:

This measurement is only a stocktaking procedure. It says nothing about the reasons for the status, and if there is a deficit where one has to begin to balance it out (intake, absorption, transportation or utilization of the vital substances).

Expert Interpretation and Recommendation --
Analyses of the Need for Nutritive Substances

Difficulties in the evaluation of the analyses

Within the normal range of such analyses, the particular circumstances of the athlete are not taken into account.
The values in the normal range (of a blood test or hair mineral analysis) represent the average of samples sent to laboratories in Germany (and thus, usually from sick people) and follow the recommendation of the DGE (German Dietetic Association).

The values published by this association (www.dge.de) only portray the minimum that a normal mortal being needs in order to avoid a deficiency.

But the need is greater if there are individual factors such as stress, the effects of environmental pollution, intensive training, illness, alcohol, nicotine, etc.

Even medical doctors specializing in sports medicine remain silent when it comes to the precise optimal levels of the individual.

One needs objective results. The best would be a holistic, naturopathic interpretation.
Influencing factors such as the personal life situation, dietary behavior, and, above all, athletic goals should be taken into account.
Certain levels can certainly lie within the normal range but be inadequate for a competition lasting several hours, and result in a limitation of performance.

Note:

I am not recommending specific products or manufacturers, as people can react differently to a given product.

In addition, receptors can change in the course of time, and with them their effects.
It is very difficult to get a clear picture of the market. New manufacturers are constantly entering the market, and some spend a lot of money on marketing. Some producers are only known to doctors and practitioners of alternative medicine.

In more economical products, carbon compounds are used, such as magnesium carbonate. But these cannot be absorbed as well as citrate compounds; for example, magnesium citrate.

There is also a manufacturer who offers minerals in liquid form. But the food coloring (cochineal red) contained in it is made up of killed scale insects. This food additive is permitted and designated as E-120 in Europe and GMP-73.100 in the United States.

My recommendation

First of all, you must make a decision -- do you want to self-medicate or would you prefer professional support in the analysis of your present condition?
Remember, it is not only a matter of athletic performance capacity, but also of answering the following question:

Why is there a deficiency?

-- Have I been taking in too few vital nutrients?

-- Have I been using too much up due to stress, work or sports?

-- Did the vital nutrients never reach the cell -- was the absorption interfered with (intestinal problems)?

Also, don't underestimate the effect of a lack of vitamins and/or minerals on the psyche, as well as on your performance capacity at work.

As long as you are not obviously sick, you will not be conscious of a deficit.

When I wanted to ride my hybrid bike over a 130k route for this time, I noticed after about 80k that my carbohydrate reserves were almost empty.
The effects of this: Physically -- "I can't go one more kilometer"; mentally -- "How do I get home now?"

I bought myself a kilogram of bananas, and after two minutes my mood improved greatly, I became more optimistic, and after ten minutes I could feel power in my legs again and rode the rest of the way.

On a daily basis, deficits usually make themselves known much more subtly. And, indeed, so subtly, that one doesn't notice them, and does not undertake anything to even them out.

Unfortunately, it is not so easy to answer the question about supplementing the diet with yes or no:

How, for instance, does a lack of selenium or zinc make itself known?
Or should I just take something, without knowing whether I have a deficit?
The pharmacy would be happy to have a regular customer … .

After making the decision (self-medication or professional assistance) get yourself -- if you decide to self-medicate -- information about preparations or individual nutrients (that is, the amount of active ingredients, sweeteners, sugar, colorings, preservatives, …), take these, and note what effect they have on you.

Question grandiose marketing claims. Check to see if your personal constitution and performance capacity improve.

And, above all, rethink your decision to take a certain preparation or individual nutrient in regular intervals; for your personal, physical or athletic situation can change, and thus make an adjustment necessary.

Examples of supplementation

Minerals are best absorbed when vitamin C -- for example, in the form of citrus fruit -- is taken at the same time.

Most minerals in the food you eat are eliminated. Only a portion of them is absorbed by the intestines and transported through the blood into the cells.
One can raise the level of absorption, when one uses the ability of the mouth's mucous membrane to absorb minerals.
Therefore, either suck on the supplements or allow minerals which have been dissolved in water to remain in the mouth for a while.

Calcium

The 2:1 ratio of calcium to magnesium is important for the cells. If you take 300 mg of calcium, you should also take 150 mg of magnesium.

Important:
Don't take both at the same time. Take calcium in the morning, and magnesium in the evening. The intestines are not able to absorb large amounts all at once.

Calcium citrate is absorbed very well. Citrate bonds with the most acids in the body.

Dosage:
Calcium citrate powder is available at the pharmacy. One level teaspoon is about the same as 250 mg.

Magnesium

Magnesium lowers blood pressure somewhat, because it expands the blood vessels. It is best to take 150 mg of magnesium one hour before going to bed.

The advantage of taking magnesium citrate is that it bonds with the most acid. You can find it at the pharmacy.

One level teaspoon contains about 200 mg of magnesium.

In the form of magnesium orotate, magnesium has an even faster and higher absorption rate, but the price is about four times higher than that of magnesium citrate. In addition, orotate is a salt of orotic acid, which is extracted from the liver or spleen of sheep. So it is not vegan.

Zinc

Zinc supports the immune system.

Zinc causes a cold to last only half as long. You might want to take 50 mg of zinc per day.

Iron

A lack of iron or an unhealthy overload of iron?

Performance athletes often need iron preparations for muscle performance and endurance. There can be a need for it when performance drops quickly, the muscles are weak or get "hung over".

Before taking iron, you should first have the stores of iron (ferritin) and the hemoglobin levels checked.

Men and older people often feel tired due to too much iron.

L-carnitine (needed for sports and when you are under stress)

L-carnitine is an amino acid / neurotransmitter. It is needed in order to carry fatty acids for the production of energy to the muscle cells. There it burns the acids in the preparation of energy (ATP).
The human body forms L-carnitine in the liver, kidneys and in the brain.
The following substances are required for its production: the amino acids methionine and lysine, the vitamins C, B3, B6, and iron.
"Normal eaters" take in carnitine when they consume meat.

Methionine and lysine are essential amino acids and must, therefore, be gotten from food.
Methionine is contained in soy, broccoli, peas, Brussels sprouts, rice and other foods.
Lysine is contained in soy, beans, peas, lentils, etc.

Using individual supplements for endurance sports is highly controversial.
Doing so is supposed to guarantee a better turnover of fatty acids by activating metabolism.
Incidentally, so far no study has shown that L-carnitine from preparations ever gets to the mitochondria in order to fulfill its function there. The bottleneck of lypolysis (mobilization of fatty acids for the preparation of energy) is a process in which L-carnitine is not involved at all.
Only the amount in the blood is raised by L-carnitine products. But this L-carnitine is excreted in the urine.

A high dosage through preparations increases the risk of the body's own L-carnitine production being stopped.

Verified advantages of L-carnitine: strengthening of the immune system, slowing down the aging process, improving liver function.

Sources: 25-1

Coenzyme Q10

Coenzyme Q10 is a vitamin-like substance that is found in almost all our body cells. There are especially high concentrations of Q10 in the cells of the liver, heart, kidneys and pancreas.

The most important functions are:

-- Antioxidative effect (protection against oxidative stress)

-- Regeneration of vitamin E and vitamin C

-- Plays an important role in energy metabolism

The human body is able to produce Q10 itself, though less with increasing age.
Q10 is present in food, but in very small amounts. It is mostly found in soy beans, walnuts and almonds.

Coenzyme Q10 is used in particular to strengthen the cardiovascular system and general vital functions.
Q10 has also been shown to be effective in the treatment of various other diseases.

Some athletes take Q10 to raise their general energy and performance levels. It has not been shown to be effective in helping already healthy people.

Selected Amino Acids

Some sports and dietary consultants recommend consuming gelatin (in the form of capsules or as a drink) in order to make protein available for the regeneration of bones and joints. This is also supposed to prevent over-straining.

The amino acids glycine and proline are also found in these gelatin products. These amino acids are important components of connective tissues. A strengthening effect on bones and joints is ascribed to them.

In principle, there is no reason to object to the recommendation of these amino acids, but why is only gelatin recommended?

A product, which is made out of pigskin, cattle skin and the bones of pigs and cattle? Or to be more precise, why do such consultants support the marketing of slaughtering wastes?

Are there alternatives to these?

What are alternative sources of the amino acids glycine and proline?

Among these are soy beans and products made from them (100 g of soy protein contains about 4.8 g of glycine and 6.2 g of proline). These amino acids are also found in other foods, among them wheat, barley, oats, peanuts and hazelnuts.

Source: 25-2

Also, when you eat soy products you are getting **all** of the essential amino acids and important secondary plant substances like isoflavones.

Genistein -- one of the isoflavones -- has an established positive role in creating bone tissue.

Studies Concerning Vegan Nutrition

Fontana L, Shaw JL, Holloszy JO, Villareal DT. Low bone mass in subjects on a long-term raw vegetarian diet.

Source 26: Archives of Internal Medicine

A recent study (2005) at the Washington University School of Medicine, St. Louis, USA yielded astonishing results.
Although the vegans studied had a lower bone mass in the hips and lumbar vertebrae, their joints and bones were still strong and solid.

This was traced back to the fact that the vegans had a different physical make-up due to their diet, causing the typical symptoms of bone loss and breaks to be absent.

In addition, the vegans had stronger immune systems, a lower BMI and a lower risk of breast cancer and cancer of the prostate gland.

Vegan proteins may reduce risk of cancer, obesity, and cardiovascular disease by promoting increased glucagon activity.
ND=ME10687887 MEDLINE (ME90)

Source 27: Medical hypotheses

Vegan proteins can reduce the risk of cancer, obesity and cardiovascular disease by increasing the production of glucagon.

Soy protein and other vegan proteins contain more non-essential amino acids than most animal products. The result of this is an increased production of glucagon and the inhibition of insulin production.
The lower insulin production is brought about by the high fiber content and low amount of saturated fatty acids usually found in a vegan diet.

Vegan proteins aid in weight loss, reduce IGF-1 activity and prevent the development of cancer.

The risk of certain "western" diseases is reduced by vegan nourishment. It also has been shown in clinical studies to be effective in preventing arthritis of the joints. Low fat vegan nutrition protects against cancer in connection with insulin resistance, and especially breast, colon and prostate cancer. The consumption of animal products has the opposite effect -- it can increase IGF-1 activity.

A note about IGF (insulin-like growth factors): In various cell culture studies it was determined that IGF-1 divides cells in the colon and prostate. IGF does its damage by taking over the regulation of cells and promoting tumors.

Sources: 27-1: (among others) http://www.milchlos.de/milos_0406g.htm

Water / Drinking

Water plays an important role in the orderly progression of life-essential chemical conversions and body functions; that is, for health in general.

A few of the tasks that water performs in the human organism:

The building block of our cells

Together with proteins water forms the fundamental substance of our cells, in which all of the other building blocks are present either in a dissolved state or already formed. This means that all the cells of our bodies are only able to function when they get enough water.

Solvent

Substances important for the organism are present in body fluids in dissolved form.

Means of transportation

Nutrients, as well as the body's own substances -- the products of metabolism, are carried to their destinations by blood plasma.

Regulation of body heat

As sweat, water is involved in this process.

When the muscles are at work, chemical energy (ATP -- adenosine triphosphate) is converted into mechanical energy and heat.

The degree of effectiveness of the muscular system is relatively low at 25 -- 30%. The remainder of the energy is "lost" as heat. When we move we become warm.

During intensive physical activity the body is forced to release the heat that has been produced by sweating, in order to avoid dangerous overheating of the organism (excessive elevation of body temperature).
Thus, if you are involved in sports, you will sweat.
Sweating does not have to be a sign of poor conditioning. On the contrary, if you are well trained for endurance sports, you can sweat well. Sweating is essential for the regulation of the organism's heat, so that body temperature doesn't rise to a dangerous level, which could lead to heat stroke.

Why is it that many athletes lose significantly more body fluid during sports activities than they replace by drinking (willingly become dehydrated)?

Is it because of fluids not being available while they are training, or not being conscious of the fact that they need fluids?

The amount and the frequency of drinking are not determined by physiological signals from the body, which tell the brain when it is time to drink. Rather, this is determined by what kinds of liquids are readily available, what we have learned from coaches, other athletes, and our parents regarding drinking while practicing sports, as well as by numerous other factors.

The loss of fluids occurs not only during the summer, but also in the winter. But we are less able to sense that we need fluids when it is cold out, and many runners don't drink anything while training or competing during the winter.
I have observed many times that even experienced runners did not drink anything while competing over 30k in the winter.

The warning signal we receive when body fluid loss reaches 2% is thirst.
You should drink something then at the latest. It is better to drink before that time, for it takes a while for the water to reach the places where it is needed. The body absorbs water through the small intestine. Drinks consumed must leave the stomach before water absorption can begin.

By the time that we become aware of thirst, we have already sacrificed some performance capacity.

Why?

Less body fluid in the blood plasma (lessening of blood volume) leads to decreased circulation, interferes with the transportation and provision of oxygen, and to a slowing down of the removal of metabolic refuse -- above all in the legs and arms.

Therefore it is important to drink water regularly in training as well as in competition (the amount depends upon the intensity of the sport and the weather conditions).
The healthy adult should normally drink 2 liters of liquids (2.1 quarts) per day when he/she is not involved in sports (recommendation: 30ml per kilogram of body weight). The loss of fluids through sports must be compensated for, in addition.
The most important and effective drink is **non-carbonated water.**

What happens when you drink too little?

The consequences are malaise, headaches, fatigue, nervousness, a drop in performance level as well as many other symptoms. Usually people are not aware of the cause.
And sometimes thirst is misinterpreted to be hunger.

Recommendation

-- You should drink ¼ to ½ liters of water before a training session or competition.

-- While your body is being stressed you should drink small amounts in short intervals, for example, 200 to 250 ml every 10 to 15 minutes.

-- If you take in a pinch of salt the water will be absorbed more quickly by the intestines.

-- In competition you should also add carbohydrates (for example, maltodextrin), about 60-80 grams per liter.
   See the section on competition diet for further information regarding maltodextrin.

-- Fruit juices and soft drinks are not suitable for making up for a loss of fluid quickly (absorption is delayed).

Source: 32

My Vegan Sports Diet

What I require of vegan nutrition for sports:

-- It should taste good to me

-- It should be healthy for me

-- It should go down well

-- It should provide me the nutrients that I need now

-- It should supply me with maximum energy for competition

-- It should refill my stores quickly after an event

What have my experiences been?

About eating right before training

I eat nothing before training. Never, no matter what amount of training I am planning, whether running 50k or swimming 15k!

Why?

In the case of a long training session, fat metabolism has to be trained.
That means: teaching the body not only to access the easily available glycogen reserves, but also the fat reserves. By doing this you will have more energy during competition, and for a longer period of time.
Of course, this is usually a process which one is unaccustomed to, and thus a laborious task for the body.

Three additional pre-conditions for making fat metabolism training easier:

-- Training on the aerobic level

-- Long training sessions

-- The body's own production of the hormone glucagon (not to be confused with glycogen -- store of carbohydrates in the muscles and liver).

Glucagon regulates carbohydrate metabolism in the liver.
Glucagon is produced for the purpose of raising the blood sugar level, as an answer to the body cells' need for sugar. Glucagon is thus the opponent of insulin and is produced in the pancreas.

The production of glucagon is stimulated when you eat protein in solid or liquid form.
That is why I have a drink of soy protein before long training sessions.

Not eating before and during training also serves to empty the muscles' glycogen stores as much as possible.
This stimulates the organism to fall back increasingly on fats for its energy supply.

At the same time, after such a training session the body will try to enlarge the glycogen depots in the musculature (see also the section on a Saltin diet as preparation right before an event).

A Brief Summary:

The ability to increase endurance is, for the most part, brought about the "training" of fat metabolism.

This training is accelerated by the production of glucagon by the body.

This hormone is produced when the concentration of glucose in the blood falls, or by an increase of the concentration of amino acids in the blood.

I achieve both when I don't ingest any carbohydrates before or during training, but rather, valuable protein (soy protein).

Source 28:
Book: Fundamentals of Biochemistry and Pathological Chemistry

Training Diet

This is actually a continuation of the previous paragraph.
While training, I want to "train in" the metabolism of fats, and thus never eat any food.

I also don't drink the isotonic drinks which are praised so much in advertising but contain sugar, or cola, energy drinks or apple juice mixtures.

Just to remind you:

Glucagon is produced as the glucose concentration in the blood goes down.
But drinks or foods containing sugar or carbohydrates prevent this from happening!

Therefore: If you want to optimize your training and achieve rapid progress in your endurance, then ignore the advertising slogans, save your money and only drink water (with a pinch of salt)!
And, above all, don't listen to athletes who tell you that these drinks helped them maintain speed even at the end of a training session.
Of course, it is true that consuming carbohydrates which enter the blood quickly will increase performance capacity.
But that has absolutely nothing to do with the purpose of training.

The after-training diet

Eat regular food after a light or moderate training session.
After a very long run, or a long swimming session, I drink soy protein and about a half hour later a meal rich in carbohydrates (with a medium to high glycemic index).

The Saltin Diet
The last week before an event

This diet serves to prepare you immediately before a competition, specifically, during the last 6 days.

The goal is to achieve a glycogen store which exceeds the normal maximum.

In this, we take advantage of the body's ability to "super-compensate".

On the sixth, fifth and fourth days before the event I only eat foods which consist almost exclusively of protein (for example, tofu, soy sprouts).

On the sixth and fifth days I train on a low level. This training, together with the protein diet, serves to empty the glycogen store almost completely.

On the days remaining before the event I eat mostly carbohydrates. Now the body reacts by storing increased amounts of glycogen. This will be available to me while competing.

One thing is clear: This method requires a lot of discipline, especially on the sixth day before the competition.

Additionally, discomfort can set in due to hunger, even after eating. But by the fifth and fourth days my body has adjusted and everything runs smoothly.

Note:

This diet only makes sense during this time period and in this context. It does not promote good health or help with training over a longer period of time in a different context!

Sixth day (before event)	Monday	Training: intermediate level Diet: Only protein
Fifth day	Tuesday	Training: low level Diet: Only protein
Fourth day	Wednesday	No Training Diet: Only protein
Third day	Thursday	No Training Diet: Focus on carbohydrates
Second day	Friday	No Training Diet: Focus on carbohydrates
First day	Saturday	No Training Diet: Focus on Carbohydrates
	Sunday	<u>Competition</u>

What to eat immediately before a competition

Early start time, or competition lasting up to 4 hours: no food or just bananas.

Late start time, or competition longer than 4 hours: millet with vegetables -- at least 2 hours before the start.

Eating during a competition

I also like to experiment with in-race diet, and allow myself to be guided by my own perception of my body.

-- No nourishment is needed in short events like the
   half-marathon.

-- Bananas should suffice for a marathon.

-- Ultra-distances or the Ironman Triathlon.
A continuous intake of carbohydrates is important in order to make possible a high level of available energy. I have had very good experiences with millet and millet biscuits, regardless of whether I am competing in a 24-hour race, the Ironman or the Lake Zurich Swim.

I was able to continue the races right after eating, as millet goes down well and is easily digestible. At 71, its glycemic index is relatively high and points to the fact that the carbohydrates are being absorbed quite quickly by the body.

At 60-80%, millet is rich in carbohydrates, contains 6-20% protein, including numerous essential amino acids and 1-6% fat. With 9mg/100g, millet contains the most iron among the common types of grain. (Only quinoa contains more iron).

Maltodextrin as a liquid alternative to nutrients in solid form such as bananas, millet or rice during competition

Maltodextrin is a white, water-soluble, odorless and nearly tasteless powder used for the energy enrichment of food.
It is a mixture of glucose saccharides and is normally obtained from cornstarch.

Maltodextrins are by definition carbohydrates with a dextrose equivalent (DE) between 5 and 20 (differing lengths of the glucose molecules).
If the DE is greater than 20 one is speaking of a glucose syrup.

The maltodextrin normally sold is maltodextrin 19 (available, for example, at the pharmacy). It is a rather short-chained maltodextrin mixture; maltodextrin 6 is long-chained.

How fast and how long are these maltodextrins effective?

Maltodextrin 19 takes effect after 10-15 minutes, and the effect lasts about 30 minutes.
The nutrients in maltodextrin 19 are absorbed more rapidly, and the dosages can be adjusted more precisely.
Maltodextrin 6 takes 2 hours to have an effect.
Therefore, I recommend against using maltodextrin 6.

Dosage:
60-80 grams in one liter of water.
Add a few pinches of cooking salt.

I advise you not to use energy drinks or power-gel

They make sugar carbohydrates available, which enter the blood rapidly in order to raise the performance level, but after just a short time the effect is gone.

My opinion concerning this is quite clear: Doing this only ignites a fire fed by straw, and after a couple of kilometers you will reach for the next gel capsule in order to maintain the same performance level.

The refined sugar burdens the intestines as well as the rest of the body. We are dealing not only with the time during competition, but also with the preparation for it.

You should test the competition nourishment, so that, in so far as possible, you will not experience a big surprise. All kinds of athletes have stomach problems with the gels.

I have never taken these products. In my observations of other athletes over short and long distances, including marathons, I have come to the conclusion that they are trying to compensate for a lack of training by taking them.

It is important to ingest carbohydrates in high intensity, long races. But you do not have to rely upon energy drinks or gels -- there are more healthy alternatives.

Drinking during competition

-- Water with a pinch of salt.

-- Soy protein as a drink while doing ultra-long-distance races or the Ironman.

> The absorption of the amino acids found in liquid soy protein reduces protein catabolism (removal of metabolic products for the purpose of detoxification of the body and for obtaining energy) and shortens regeneration time.

138

Post-competition nutrition

Immediately afterwards: a drink of soy protein and then easily digestible carbohydrates, like bananas or millet.

Later on: emphasis on carbohydrate-rich meals, in order to refill the glycogen store.
Depending on the length of the event (and also the strain and weather conditions) I take minerals and algae as a dietary supplement.

Vegan Recipes for Endurance Athletes -- such as, millet biscuits for competition -- will be provided in another book to be published early in 2006.

Growth Hormone (STH/GH)

(STH = Somatotropic Hormone)

Different amino acids such as arginine, ornitihine, lysine, glycine, glutamine and tryptophan stimulate the release of growth hormones from the pituitary gland.

The growth hormone acts anabolically (therefore promotes muscle growth, for example) in the following organs: -- bones
                                                         -- muscles
                                                         -- liver

That means, in these organs it leads to an increased absorption of amino acids and processing of them.
In addition, STH raises the blood sugar level and has a lipolytic effect on the fat cells -- breaks down fat.

STH production is stimulated by a low blood glucose level. But a diet with a high glycemic index disrupts the release of STH.

Source 29: CO'MED Magazine, Basiswissen Biochemie mit Pathobiochemie

What does this mean for an athlete?

Like its name says, growth hormone causes growth (of muscles, for example) and aids in the breaking down of fat. Both of these things support an athlete in his effort to expand performance capacity.
By stimulating growth, this hormone also slows the aging process (more of it is produced during puberty).

How is the pituitary gland stimulated to produce STH?

-- By a lower blood sugar level -- especially in the evening.

-- By processes that use up energy, for example, endurance sports.

-- By (for example) liquid soy protein (Soy protein contains all of the essential amino acids. 1 tablespoon in one half glass of water), taken right before going to bed. This is the best time, because the most STH is produced during sleep.

As the effects differ among individuals (some think they wake up more refreshed), I recommend trying this on different days.
Observe whether and which beneficial effects it has.

After an evening training session, taking a soy protein drink (and avoiding carbohydrates) is <u>not</u> advisable, as STH causes a reduction in the absorption of glucose.
But immediately after training, loading up the carbohydrate store is of the utmost importance (for the regeneration and readying of energy for the next training session).

Note:

In different places in this book I recommend soy protein in powder form.

When you are purchasing it, I recommend that you see that as little as possible or none at all of the following ingredients are contained in it: flavorings, sugar, other sweeteners and carbohydrates.

The Fundamentals of Endurance Sports

All aerobic sports are endurance sports, including running, swimming, cycling, cross-country skiing, in-line skating, walking, etc.

The term "aerobic" means that there is no oxygen deficit while the sport is being practiced. So, at least as much oxygen is taken in as is used up.

Advantages and health benefits of regular training (using running as an example):

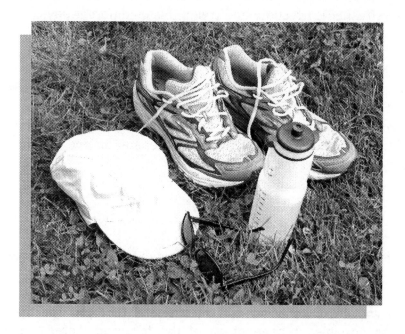

-- Improvement of breathing by expanding lung capacity and, along with it, endurance.

-- Improvement of heart performance. The heart is also a muscle. Through endurance training, it becomes stronger and larger, learning to push more blood through the body with fewer beats. That takes some strain off of it as well.
In addition, the risk of heart disease drops by about one-half.

-- Moderate endurance training lowers "bad" cholesterol (low-density lipoproteins = LDL) in the body. It also raises "good" cholesterol (high-density lipoproteins = HDL). This reduces the risk of arteriosclerosis (the build-up of plaque), heart attacks, strokes and high blood pressure.

-- It decelerates the aging process and strengthens the immune system, especially when you train outside and in any kind of weather.

-- Through this you become better balanced, and more resistant to stress. The good mood endurance training puts you in lasts for a long time. You can handle stress better, because stress hormones are released more slowly and in smaller concentrations.

-- You sleep better, more deeply and are more refreshed when you wake up.

-- Your bone density increases, lowering the risk of osteoporosis.

-- The increase of oxygen available to you improves your concentration and memory.

The ideal weight

Many of the diets advertised in magazines make use of the dehydrating effect of certain foodstuffs.
This does lower weight, but not a single ounce of body fat is lost!

Usually people quit the diet after a short time, for the selection of foods is not sufficient or healthy in the long run, or cannot be handled mentally.
This leads to their putting all of the weight lost back on.
Such yo-yo dieting merely teaches the body to use the calories consumed more efficiently.
The need for exercise and sports is also reduced, out of pure frustration, among other things. The body starts storing even more fat, in order to prepare for the next fasting time (spring diet).
Less exercise means that basal metabolism is reduced even more.
The result is continuous weight gain.
Every year the entire procedure begins again. They look in the mirror -- I'm overweight! They decide on a diet, and only become frustrated when the starting weight is exceeded all over again.

Some people do this all of their lives.

Only regular endurance training can elevate basal metabolism (energy used while the body is at rest).

Assuming no changes in diet, the result is that you lose weight continuously. When you are first starting the program, it could happen that the building of muscles will cause your weight to remain the same.
But the deciding factor is that the fat component of your weight has been reduced.

If, in addition, you improve your diet (see the chapter on vegan nutrition) the fat cushions shrink drastically and permanently.

Then your body weight will reach its ideal level. This weight level is synonymous with improved health, fitness, vitality, success in competition and improved performance capacity.

Notes regarding endurance sports

Although it would be nice, endurance sports are not a panacea for all possible illnesses. But they do substantially reduce factors which contribute to disease.

Meanwhile, it has been established that people who are out of shape are more likely to have a heart attack when they exert themselves too much than are those who train regularly.

In a study it was shown that the total risk of sudden death due to a coronary infarct is 60% less in people who are very active physically than in those who are less active.
Exercising reasonably and seeing the doctor regularly reduces the risk of dying suddenly of a heart attack.

Recommendations by doctors:

Patients who practice endurance sports regularly and suffer from asthma or bronchitis improve their lung capacity and suffer less from lack of oxygen.
Endurance sports are a part of treatment for most lung diseases.

Source: 30

Over 50% of deaths are caused by heart attack or cardiovascular disease.

90% of the risk factors for these diseases can be influenced by exercise:

blood fats, blood pressure, blood sugar/diabetes, smoking, overweight, lack of movement.

Only 10% can not be influenced: age, gender, family history.

Sufficient moderate (aerobic) sports activity (3 x 30 minutes per week) lowers blood pressure.

Brief, extremely high physical exertion (for example, anaerobic sports, intensive labor) puts an excessive burden on the body and increases the danger of a coronary event.

Source: 31

Conclusions:

-- **Endurance Sports aid health and increase vitality.**

-- **Those who are not presently training (regardless of age) should undergo a complete physical exam including cardiovascular function before beginning training.**

Training, goal-setting, training schedules

What does training mean?

Training is a planned increase in the performance capacity of the body, especially the muscles and cardiovascular system.
In this, physical efforts are repeated in a targeted manner, in order to reach a certain goal (distance, speed). Training has to be thought out on an individual basis, for it depends on the goal sought after and the body's current status.

Example:
The optimal preparation for a marathon run would be running 30-35k several times.
An increase in volume (sum of kilometers run in a week) and intensity (speed, climbs) should also be a part of this.

There are varying philosophies regarding the creation of a training plan:

First approach:

2 weeks with increasing volume and intensity (from week 1 to week 2).
After that, a week for regeneration with low volume and intensity. During the following week, training is continued with a higher volume than week 1.

Second approach:

Some people use 3 + 1 -- 3 weeks of increasing effort and then 1 week of reduced training.
This training reduction aids in regeneration and the adjustment to a higher load.

Example:

First Sequence

Week 1	Week 2	Week 3	Week 4
2 x 10k	3 x 12k	4 x 12k	3 x 10k

Second Sequence

Week 5	Week 6	Week 7	Week 8	etc.
2 x 12k	3 x 15k	4 x 15k	3 x 12k	etc.

I don't recommend any particular training regimens, as everyone has a different goal, a different physical "constitution", a different environment (job, family), and has a different route to cope with in competition (flat, hilly, spring, summer heat).

You can't get out of trying out what is beneficial in your situation.

This testing has the advantage of helping you to learn quickly what body signals to pay attention to, and to make training adjustments.

A pre-prepared training plan does provide something to cling to, but doesn't take into account your personal potential and limitations.

One of these limitations is your body's performance capacity. It needs time to adjust to the greater load being put on it.
Once a certain volume of training or velocity has been reached, the body can react to this stress with complaints -- tendons, joints, muscles, malaise, motivation, ...

This limit is entirely individual.

What can be done?

More stretching exercises, training adjustments, working through mental blocks, using another sport to even things out (cross-training), simply accepting this limit for this year, or ... .

I strongly advise you not to ignore the current performance capacity limit, because the complaints and symptoms will probably get worse and lead to an even longer forced interruption of training.

Training Fundamentals

An effective endurance training regimen is oriented toward expanding performance capacity and strengthening the cardio-vascular system.

Further aspects, such as trunk stability, mental strength or the load the joints and tendons can handle also deserve attention. But the heart and circulatory system is the area you should focus on if you desire effective endurance training.

Why?

The heart/circulatory system (cardiovascular system) supplies every cell with oxygen and nutrients. In sports, the heart in particular is responsible for providing these to the muscle cells. The higher the muscular performance level is, the harder the heart must be able to pump in order to supply the muscle cells adequately. So, the faster you run, the faster the blood must flow as it circulates.

In addition, metabolic products, hormones and waste products like carbon dioxide are carried along.

The better the cells are supplied and the faster waste is carried away, the healthier and more able to perform your body will become.

An increase in the performance capacity of the cardiovascular system is achieved by an adjustment to the increased load created by training. The heart is a muscle which changes in size, and thus in performance capacity over the course of time. The heart muscle becomes larger through regular athletic training.

That is why a well-trained endurance athlete has a lower resting heart rate than someone who doesn't train.

In the case of an endurance athlete, fewer heartbeats are needed in order to transport blood for the purpose of attaining the desired performance level.

The resting heart rate is directly proportional to heart size. In performance athletes 40 beats per minute are normal (in adults, this is best measured immediately after waking up in the morning).

In endurance athletes the pulse is usually between 50 and 60 beats per minute.

The health and performance capacity of the heart and circulatory system is the very foundation of the physical and athletic constitution.

To change the focus from sports:
It is worthwhile for every person to strive for cardiovascular health and performance capacity.
This will result in an improvement in the quality of life through vitality, fitness and health.

Here I wish to establish a link to the title of this book:
Vegan nutrition and endurance sports are two very important factors -- **perhaps the most important** -- which you can influence yourself. The heart and circulatory systems in particular profit from your doing without animal products.

How can I "train in" my heart/circulatory system in order to increase athletic performance?

Targeted endurance training trains in:

-- the heart/circulatory system

-- metabolism (for example, of fats)

-- the corresponding muscle groups

Here, there is mutual interaction:

Through running, the cardiovascular system is trained at different speeds, distances and in different training environments, taking into account your current personal situation.
This is am important point in planning your training regimen. As there are so many personal peculiarities in diet and endurance training, I recommend training your physical perception. Listen to your body to see if a change in training is called for.

In your daily life, personal "tweaking" of diet and training should have a high priority

One small example of how the one overlaps into the other:
Soy products supply all essential amino acids, and are a basis for building muscle and regenerating after a training session or competition.
The amino acids methionine and lysine, contained in soy protein, are needed for the body's own production of L-carnitine (fat metabolism/fat burning).
Additionally, soy protein promotes metabolism during long runs in "Zone 1" (to be explained later).

A performance enhancing fat metabolism makes possible noteworthy achievements in long-distance events.

Carbohydrates with a high glycemic index accelerate the building up of glycogen stores after training.

If the same carbohydrates are consumed without training, the risk of getting Type 2 Diabetes is drastically raised over the long run.

Thus it depends entirely upon your personal life and training situation, whether and how much of certain foods or training sessions are reasonable or not.

It is stated repeatedly concerning athletes that they are in good touch with their own bodies and are very intuitive. In my opinion, one cannot overstate the significance of trusting in your own intuition.

For example, there are world class swimmers who change their body positioning in training for so long that they can "feel" a slight current resistance.

Therefore, my recommendation: Open up all your senses, trust in your intuition, and also try out things that may be unconventional. That which is ideal today, could slow you down next week in training. Or vice versa.

Energy provision

An understanding of the processes involved here makes it possible for you to employ influencing factors such as training and nutrition in a targeted manner.

Glycogen is stored glucose in the muscles and liver. In an intensive training session or competition, muscular glycogen lasts for about 60-90 minutes.
The store in the liver serves to maintain a constant blood sugar level. If the supply is used up, and no carbohydrates are taken in, hypoglycemia (low blood sugar) can develop.

During a low-intensity run, first the glycogen in the liver is tapped, and then the muscle glycogen.
During a high-intensity run, the reverse is the case.

Body fat can also be changed into glucose. This chemical process takes place much more slowly, so that the use of body fat has significance in less strenuous exercise.

Energy can be obtained from glycogen and body fat in different ways:

Aerobic -- Getting energy without an oxygen deficit occurring.
A constant load of excess oxygen leads to an improvement in endurance.
This is achieved after about 30 minutes.

At low intensity, the metabolism prefers to reach for the almost inexhaustible body fat reserves.
If the tempo is increased slightly, the metabolism prefers to access the glycogen reserves.

Anaerobic -- Training in Zone 2 or at still higher speed. When to begin training at this level is dependent upon your personal performance capability.

Obtaining energy:

-- <u>with</u> lactate production, or

-- <u>without</u> the production of lactate (milk acid).

In anaerobic alactacidic metabolism, there is an oxygen deficit **and no** lactate is formed.
This is utilized in sprint training. In a run in Zone 1 sprints are carried out in Zone 2.
Suggestion 1: 200 meter distance with 10 repetitions.
Suggestion 2: 1,000 meter (1k) distance with 5 repetitions.

In between sprints, run in Zone 1 until the lactate is broken down or reduced, and the same high level of performance is achieved in the next interval.
What stands out in the anaerobic area is the increase in speed and the "enduring" of a higher tempo over a longer period of time.

Important: Observe an even tempo while training (except during interval training). This creates the greatest training effect.

Lactate elucidated: (a salt of milk acid, created in the metabolic process) --
The need for oxygen is increased when a muscle is asked to perform at a higher level. If the blood supplied does not cover this need for oxygen, lactate is created by an incomplete burning of glucose.

Training in Zone 1

The focus of endurance training should be here. The less you train, the more important it is to train a lot percentage-wise in this zone. With increasing endurance an increase in running speed is possible, as well as further training in the aerobic area.

If you are training with a pulse meter or want to: Zone 1 corresponds to 60-75% of the maximum heart rate.

In order to determine your personal MHR it will be necessary to go "all out" during a run.

Here, once again the advice:

I recommend seeing a medical doctor for a thorough physical examination before you begin endurance training, and at certain intervals afterwards. If there is a pre-existing cardiovascular condition, it is not advisable to determine your maximum heart rate by means of a run at full capacity.

I also recommend that you see a doctor if your pulse remains at MHR for a few minutes after this experiment.

It is best to carry out this experiment in the morning.

According to your performance capability, warm up more or less, then do a few short sprints, and finish with a run at maximum speed. If there is a high stairway on a mountain or in a high-rise building available to you, you could use this to achieve a full load on your heart.
An alternative would be to run 3k and sprint 400 meters as fast as you can at the end.

The heart rate for the individual training zones is calculated on the basis of this result.

The maximum heart rate cannot be used to determine your personal performance capability. It would make sense to check the MHR at long intervals in order to avoid over- or undertaxing yourself.

-- Regeneration run   up to 60% of the maximum heart rate

-- Zone 1   60-75%

-- Zone 1 / 2   75-85%

-- Zone 2   85-90/95%

-- Tempo running   over 90/95%

Zone 1

The area of fat metabolism training: Fats can only be broken down aerobically (aerobic lypolysis).

What does fat metabolism training mean?
The provision of energy takes place via the glycogen stores in the muscles and body fat. The body is accustomed to accessing the readily available glycogen supplies.

The problem is that these stores are quickly exhausted when you go long distances and/or at a high rate of speed.
That is why the body is trained to access the nearly inexhaustible body fat reserves (1kg of body fat suffices for a 100k run). In Zone 1 the glycogen supplies are conserved and a high proportion of body fat is used in providing energy.
That means that a training session in Zone 1 serves to improve endurance over long stretches.

157

How can I tell that I am in Zone 1 if I'm not using a pulse watch?
If I can converse fluently, I am in Zone 1.

Zone 2

When you are well-grounded in Zone 1, you should begin to include a run at higher speed in your training plan. This will be faster than Zone 1, and serve to increase your future competition speed.
Due to the higher intensity, the need for regeneration is greater and the following training sessions could be negatively impacted. Therefore, this training at a higher speed should not be done too often or for too long.

Suggestion:
A run of a maximum of 15k each week. It should be possible to accelerate during the last kilometer.

How can I tell if I am in Zone 2 if I'm not using a pulse watch?
If my conversation is regularly interrupted by pauses to take a breath, I am in Zone 2.

Racing speed / Competition tempo

Faster than in Zone 2. This rate includes marathon running. But in an ultra-marathon, the competitors do not normally attempt to reach this speed.

Interval training

This involves a tempo run, which takes place in Zone 2. The planning of this training session depends on your performance capacity and goal.

For example, a 200m sprint and then 1k at normal speed -- and all of this 10 times; or, a 10k run and every 500 m a 100 m sprint.

For further tempo training variations see the preceding section: Anaerobic energy preparation.

Training time in the context of preparing for an event

When there is little or no evidence to go on, it is only natural that a prognosis is difficult. If you want to participate in a competitive event, take a look at your progress during the preparatory period, and whether any sort of serious complaints or symptoms are present.

Even if it is tough for you: Don't try to force anything. So many competitions are held that deciding to participate in one at a later point in time could make very good sense.

If you are properly trained according to the above description, I recommend a preparatory period of about 3 months for a marathon, and at least 6 months for ultra-marathons or the Ironman.

In training for competition, "The athlete is made in the winter" is the saying. During this season, the foundations are laid. Someone who just "wakes up" in the spring can only become fit for events which take place in the fall.

Distribution of training time and zones

70% "Basic" training (Zone 1)

30% Tempo training with interval training/sprints, tempo runs, and performance enhancement runs (Zone 2 or faster)

Additionally:

Stretching exercises
(see chapter on Stretching Exercises)

Strengthening of the trunk muscles
(see chapter on Upper Body Exercises)

Long or fast training sessions?

"Do I have to train a lot in Zone 1, if I only take part in short races?"

-- Even then, regular Zone 1 training makes sense. The foundation is improved, and there are many health benefits.

"Does it make sense to do sprints when training for a long race?"

-- Of course it does.
   This will increase your speed in the competition.

Swimming Training

The focus of this book is on running. Despite this, I would like to cover a few aspects of swimming training, for there are many similarities between it and running training.

The most important points in common

-- The preparation of energy is identical

-- Training plan
   Short training sessions: interval training, tempo training 1-3k
   Long training sessions beginning at 5,000 meters

-- Distribution of training time
   70% Zone 1, 30% Zone 2, stretching exercises, upper body exercises

Although it is difficult for some to begin regular swimming training, I especially recommend it.

The positive effects on health, fitness and other sports are very great.
Swimming the breast stroke, however, can cause neck and knee symptoms when done intensively.

I recommend doing the crawl stroke. It strengthens the back and abdominal muscles, and in this way contributes to good running posture.
If you have a very good swimming technique, the running musculature is loosened up, it's easy on your joints (thus, swimming is ideal for overweight athletes), and the cardiovascular system is trained splendidly, which improves endurance.

Some important differences between swimming training and running training

Technique training

Due to the high amount of resistance created by the water, it is important how energy is put to use and whether the body's posture offers little resistance to the current.

Preparing for competition over long distances

In swimming, significantly more calories are used up than in running.
Part of preparation is keeping an eye on what you eat and drink: When should I eat and drink? What will set well with me?

Mental preparation -- dealing with changes in the weather, possible leg cramps, only short conversations with those accompanying you in the boat ("isolation").
Physical and mental preparation for a low water temperature in a lake or the ocean.

Fatigue due to the higher energy consumption is not to be under-estimated, nor is the lowered metabolism when you are swimming in the morning or at night.
This can be difficult to train for, if there is no suitable open water near you.

Additionally, swimming training is made all the more difficult when, for safety reasons, people are supposed to accompany you in a boat (because of boat traffic or the danger of hypothermia).

In open water competition, preparation -- especially mental preparation -- is of much greater importance than in running.

For example, in long-distance running it is not a problem to sit down for a meal or to remain standing.

In the case of a leg cramp it is possible to get rid of it by doing a stretching exercise (fortunately I have never had this experience, but have seen it happen to other runners).

Time planning for competition preparation can also differ

In the summer of 2006 I plan to swim the Crossing of the Straits: **www.beltquerung.de**

Through the Baltic Sea from Denmark to Fehmarn island, 21k by air (depending on the currents the organizer assumes 25k), water temperature about 15-20 degrees Celsius (59-68 degrees Fahrenheit).

I will swim without a neoprene suit and merely allow myself to put on a little fat.

Thus, adjusting to the cold is very important to me.

I began the necessary preparation 9 months before the swim.

In November, I put a 300 liter rain barrel in the garden, and will take a dip in it regularly all winter long, staying in it as long as possible, in order to get used to cold water.

In addition, the program includes training over long distances in cold water (a river or a lake).

Running for Novices

Regardless of your reason for beginning to run, it is best to start with regular training.

It is especially important in the beginning to train slowly and cautiously.
With growing experience, it will become easier and easier in the future to bring your physical and mental performance capability into harmony with your running goals.
This assumes a realistic self-appraisal.
More precisely: You will need to sense body signals and pay attention to them.
In other words, be honest with yourself!

So don't put additional pressure to succeed on yourself, just because other runners are passing you or you want badly to participate in a certain event.

What would you like to accomplish with running?

-- Do something for your health?

-- Lose weight?

-- Raise your performance capacity?

According to what your main motivation is, you should carefully examine your present condition and situation (physically, mentally and time-wise).

I recommend that you make a check-list regarding your goals (amount of training, competitions, speed) and to go through it item by item.

Physically

Overweight, advanced age or unhealthy lifestyle (diet, alcohol, nicotine)?
In these cases I recommend seeking a doctor's advice before starting to train.
If you are overweight, it is often advisable to start with an endurance sport that is easy on your joints, like swimming or bicycling.
Only start running after you have lost the proper amount of weight.

Even if you can "see yourself" in a marathon run, check regularly whether running progress is good for you and your body.

Mentally

In what kind of weather or at what temperature do you want to run?
Where do you want to run? In the beginning, it is advisable to choose routes that are as flat as possible -- do not attempt to run up a mountain!

Time-wise

When, how often and for how long do you want to run?
In the morning, evening or only on Sunday?
What do your family and friends have to say about your decision to train?
There will be training sessions after which you will feel fit and energetic, but there will be some that will cause you to need peace and quiet.

Starting to train -- some recommendations

-- Seek out a pleasant training environment for yourself: forest, lake, park ... .

-- Don't eat anything for at least 2 hours before training.
   Fruit is o.k. one hour before beginning.

-- Drink a lot of water before the training session.

-- A training session with other runners is supportive, as long as they start out slowly and then run at an even pace.

-- In the beginning, set small goals for yourself. It could suit you to run 1-3k at one time.
   Or run for 5 minutes, walk for 3 minutes and finish up with a 5 minute run.
   Make sure that your regimen makes you feel good and doesn't overstress you.

This approach will help you more than trying to run 10k and ending the run prematurely, exhausted, frustrated and with pains in your sides.

If you have already been training for a while

-- Increase the amount of training at the speed that is comfortable for you. It is better to exercise slowly but continuously.

-- Give more attention to stretching exercises after training and also on non-training days.

-- Don't forget the importance of body posture.
   Which posture feels good and which causes symptoms?

-- Consider whether another sport or other fitness exercises could "round-off" your training (cross-training).
   (Yoga, strength training, …).

-- Strengthening torso musculature makes running easier – especially on longer courses. This is where your leverage for running comes from. Energy originates in the trunk.
   This is true of both running and swimming.
   See also the chapters on **Running Style** and **Upper Body Exercises**.

How often should I train?

Three times a week would be ideal, with a day of rest in between each session.
If you occasionally can only train for one day, it doesn't matter. The main thing is that you stick with it and run three times again the following week.

Simulating an Ultra-run
(or a shorter distance)

If you are training for an ultra-marathon or are considering attempting one sometime in the future, here is a training suggestion.

If you are training for a half-marathon or marathon, a reduction in the extent of training suggested here will be just as helpful for you.

I will be discussing primarily the principles here. It will be necessary for you to make adjustments as fits your particular performance level and the goal you have set for yourself.

Simulation of an ultra-run: the procedure

My past history: When I made the decision to participate in a 24 hour run, I thought about what kind of training I would need for this.

For the first 100k run, I ran 100k or more per week many times. Actually I should have trained more for the 24 hour run.

But where should I get the time from, and how would my body handle the stress, especially since I still wanted to train for swimming and triathlon competitions?

So it was time to implement a new form of training.

The requirements were clear:
-- A simulation of an ultra-run, in order to prepare myself mentally and physically for a very long distance.

-- Not to put too much stress on my tendons and joints.

-- To really empty out my glycogen stores, in order to take advantage of the super-compensation effect (I elaborate on this in the section on super-compensation).

168

Therefore, I carried out the following training procedure:

-- On Saturday mornings at 5:00 I ran a route which I had measured with a bicycle odometer. It ended at home. 5.6k at a speed of 5:30 (minutes per kilometer) in a maximum time of 30 minutes.

-- Then I didn't run for a half hour, occupying myself with "everyday things": cleaning, shopping, vacuuming … .

-- After that, I repeated this cycle of 30 minutes of running and 30 minutes of not running 8 times.

-- This way, I ran 45k, and was home for lunch at 12:30 pm.

Pre-conditions

Before the first or second round I drink soy protein in order to stimulate the production of glucagon. By doing so, I raise the proportion of fat-supplied energy as high as possible. I also conserve the glycogen supply, improving endurance.

I only drink water before the run, during the run and the non-running time.

NO fruit, carbohydrates or drinks containing them.

Through activities while not running I prevent my metabolism from sinking too low.

You should never lie down or take a total break.

Background data

-- Duration, physically: I run in Zone 1. The glycogen stores are almost emptied out in the course of these cycles (therefore, I am also doing things while not running).

-- Duration, mentally: I trained for 7.5 hours altogether. There is no comparison between running 30k in one stretch, or for 7.5 hours and feeling very hungry all the way to the end.

-- Distance: 45k, but the stress on the tendons and joints is 50% less (as if I had run about 25k in one stretch). So it is really easy on these parts of the anatomy.

My personal experience

During round 6 of my first simulation I was thinking, "Where is my energy, why am I constantly thinking of taking a walking break? I've only run 33k."
It was true that I had only run 33 kilometers, but the fatigue and the duration (over 5 hours) had an effect.

What typically happens

Round 1: I am not really comprehending the fact that I am running, and ask myself why I am running at 5:00 am, when I won't be running between 5:30 and 6:00.

Rounds 2-4: normal running.

Rounds 5-6: I become distinctly aware of the reason for this type of training. The mental challenge increases.

Rounds 7-8: The deep emptying of the glycogen stores continues. At first, it was not so easy to maintain speed.

After the eighth round I become aware that I have finished the routine again. I have improved my endurance and mental strength.

Because I nearly empty the glycogen stores, I have almost completely simulated a real ultra-marathon run.

The physical and emotional low points were brought about by the dwindling glycogen supplies, increasing hunger and the strain, both physical and time-wise.

I had to cope with this, and during the last 2 months before the 24 hour run I developed a routine by means of the repetitions.

The progress made in training was made evident by the fact that I was able to maintain speed easily and even increase it during the last rounds.

Despite the demands of training I felt fit and mentally strengthened.

> After I had done 5 such simulations, I ran 50k in one stretch including 700 meters of climbing.
>
> After this run I was still fit and in a good mood. And, above all: I knew that I was mentally and physically prepared for the 24 hour run.

Recommendation

If you should consider this kind of training, experiment in order to find out how you would best begin it: mornings at 7:00, 4 rounds; or at 9:00, 3 rounds; or 8 rounds right away in order to acquire concrete experience immediately.

And the process of learning and trying out new ideas goes on ...

In the meantime, I have asked myself a few questions:

"How would it work if I used the racing bike with the roller-trainer set at a very low speed during these "non-running times"?

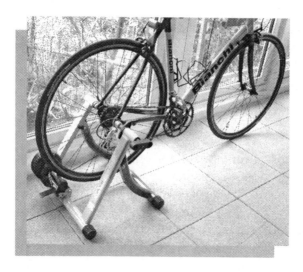

In the winter it is possible to keep training yourself in the fundamentals by doing this -- without putting yourself and others in danger on ice and snow.

"Wouldn't this help me make the switch from cycling to running in the triathlon, and increase cycling endurance ... ?"

"Should I do this right from the beginning, or wait until the last rounds ... ?"

It appears to me that right now (at the beginning of 2006) would be a good time to look into these questions.

I will change my training and find out whether this would be an improvement.

Then I will prepare myself for a 24-hour run (May 2006) and the Ironman Triathlon (July 2006).

"... after the 24-hour run and before the Ironman I should probably change my focus when it comes to intensity. Medium to high intensity (Zone 1) on the roller-trainer (30 minutes), and during non-cycling times running at low intensity ... ?"

I am mentioning these questions, because they reflect my training philosophy:

Is there something that could be improved, even though other athletes haven't yet tried something like this?

What types of training are correct for me, and which ones would be best two months from now?

Running Style

Is there a running style that is ideal for ALL runners, or should every runner keep his or her own style?
In observing elite runners, and the effects of body posture on their body structure, it cannot be overlooked that they have certain things in common.

In everyday life, body posture also plays an important role. Many people suffer from back pain or tension when they work bent over their desks or do manual labor in a bent-over position.

In running, this kind of strain also plays a role. If you run with a "round back" for a short while, you will be just as exhausted as if you had spent all day bent over a desk.
So running style has a great effect on how you feel during training and on the time you turn in after a competition.

The most important goals in running:

    -- it should be fun

    -- it should be healthy

    -- you want to be fast during an event

To put all three points together: It is important to be constantly checking your body posture and correcting it when necessary.

But how can you check your own body posture, and how can you make it ideal?

The usual scenario ...

You go and buy yourself some running shoes and start running. You've been running since you were a kid, so you don't have to think about the "proper" way to run.

Why should you want to learn how to run? For heaven's sake, you are already 20, 30 or 40 years old!

Usually no one will inform you that there is an ideal running style that must be learned (aside from a few people with natural talent). It also doesn't always happen that people get feedback in their running clubs or groups.
Most of the time the leader will have developed his/her own style, and doesn't feel that it is worth talking about with other runners.

Training conversations usually concern the amount of training, events or personal matters.

Why is it so seldom that people pay attention to running style, and how to acquire the ideal one?
Isn't it perceived to be important, or don't people want to face something that could be unpleasant or difficult?!

I am being serious here. You need a certain amount of humility to face the facts: Your own running style is not ideal; and, even in something as banal as running appears to be, you will have some things to learn.

> If you don't know anyone who is qualified to give you feedback, run by show windows frequently, using them as a mirror in which to look at your own running style at different speeds.

What are the characteristics of a healthy body posture and high performance capability in running?

An erect upper body puts the proper stress on the spine.
Only if your upper body is vertical can you swing your arms parallel to the direction you are running in and not across the front of your body.
This will help you to run much better.

In order to hold the upper body up you need a well developed torso musculature.
These strong muscles will make running easier -- especially on longer courses. These trunk muscles provide the leverage which makes you able to run. Your energy is transferred from here.

A weak upper body and/or poor posture cause, among other things, faster fatigue, slower speed (shortness of strides/frequency of strides) and possibly wear and tear due to poor body posture.

The next important points concern the legs and feet.

Stride length and frequency are determined by leg movements and the leg muscles which are employed in them.

In moving your legs you should ensure that your heels are brought up as high as possible.
It is also important to lift up your knees.

Read on for a few more pages, and you will find exercises for training the muscles needed for doing these things. This will make it easier to acquire the running style I have described.

How should I put my feet down?

On the balls of my feet, the arches or the heels?
Even the experts have differing opinions regarding this.
Whom should I believe -- and why?

How would you run if you were not wearing shoes?

Try running barefoot at varying speeds and note the different effects on your body.
It would be ideal if you could conduct this test on a variety of surfaces, such as grass or pavement.

What makes your body feel the best?

Slow speed or walking:

Do you find it to be most pleasant when you plant your whole foot down on the surface?

Medium speed:

Do you find it to be most pleasant when you run on the balls and middle part of your feet?

Fast speed – sprinting

Do you find it to be most pleasant when you run on your forefeet?
(forefoot = balls of the foot, not the toes)

Running on your heels causes quite a shock to your body -- to the knees, for example. The faster you go the worse it becomes.
The thick heels of running shoes are supposed to reduce this, but a strain (which is preventable) is still present.

In principle, then, a correct running style is quite simple. (There are other things to pay attention to -- but these are the most important):

Upper body erect, arms swinging parallel, raise up on your heels, and plant your feet on their balls or in the middle.
In the beginning paying attention to all of these points could get on your nerves, but after a while you will be further motivated when you notice that you are progressing.

With what you have read here in the back of your head, take a look at the running style of and general impression made by:

-- elite runners at a competition or on television,
   and

-- the faster and slower runners at an open cross-country race or city marathon -- are their running styles different?

Doing this will make it easier for you to examine your own running style and will enable you to learn the optimal running style more quickly.
Due to the fast movements it will be helpful to concentrate for a while on one part of this at a time: arm work; planting of the feet; or, the movements of the legs.

Aspects of a good running style

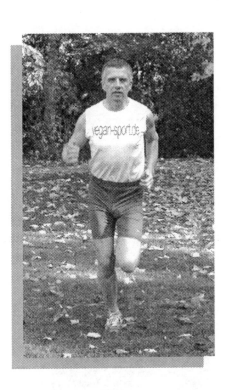

Eyes straight ahead, upper body erect, arms swinging parallel to the running direction, slight tension in the abdominal muscles.

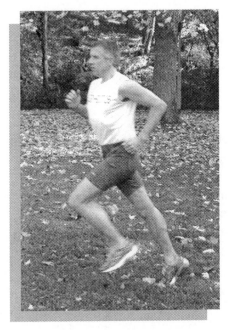

Upper body vertical, arms swing toward the front and rear, front knee lifted up, front foot planted on its balls and middle.

Two examples of body postures which do not support a runner

Short step length, "sitting" slightly, little arm swing.

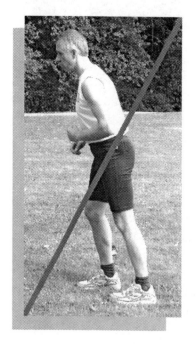

Short step length, upper body leaning toward front, arms swing in front of the body and can cause a rotation of the upper body. In addition, they prevent the runner from reaching a high speed.

Comparison of poor posture and the ideal posture

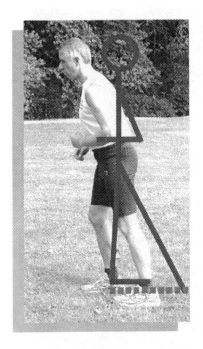 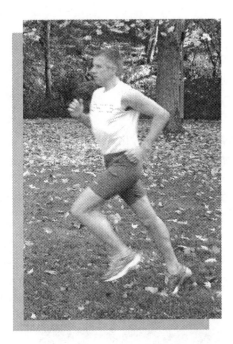

The difference between the short line (between the feet) and the long, dotted line is a greater step length.

Because you have to take thousands of steps in a competition, a greater step length means you will run faster and finish sooner.

Raising the frequency of steps will further increase your speed.

**Practicing these 2 exercises will increase
your striding rate**

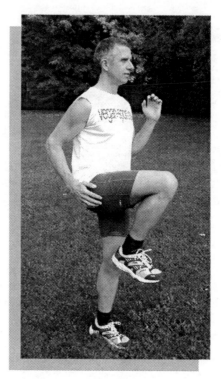

Procedure:

While standing, lift your
knees up as far as possible
in short intervals. Rapid
repetitions.
Do this for 3 minutes.

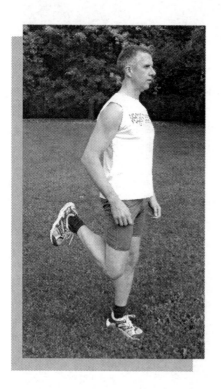

Procedure:

While standing, raise your
heels up to your buttocks
(hitting them) or as far as
possible.

Rapid repetitions.
Do this for 3 minutes.

Regeneration and Super-Compensation

There are at least as many recommendations as there are athletes concerning the proper mixture of training and regeneration.
But there are a few points of agreement that are worth taking a look at.
The deciding factor is a good feeling about your body, or self-perception.

Regeneration

By regeneration I mean the restoration of my physical performance capability. The intensity and duration of the prior athletic strain influences the need for regeneration.

Short regeneration phase
After a training session the most important thing is the re-filling of the glycogen stores in the muscles and liver, and the production of enzymes for the readying of energy. For this, primarily carbohydrates, protein and valuable fatty acids are needed.

Intermediate regeneration phase
During a training week I include one or another day without training with a goal in mind. On these days, the metabolic rebuilding processes are of the utmost importance, and the depots are filled with minerals and vitamins.

Longer regeneration phase
After a competition there is a more or less high need for regeneration, according to the duration and intensity of the event. Also, I have run out of steam mentally by the time I reach the finish line. In this phase, it is important to me to do little training and to sleep a lot.

These building-up processes lead to an improvement of performance -- the training effect. The body adjusts itself to the new endurance stress and along with that the individual performance capacity increases.

Through constantly recurring stress the body is prepared for the next training unit (or competition), and it makes available the energy needed for this.

This adjustment or endurance increase does not, however, take place in the stress stage, but rather in the regeneration phase.

1. During a training run

A walking or trotting break during an interval training session.

2. During a training week

I train three to six days per week in intensity and/or volume, in which the speed or the length of the session is increased, while exertion remains the same. Then a regeneration day follows (or between the training units).

3. Over several months

When planning for a competition, the intensity as a whole increases -- according to your training philosophy -- over 2 or 3 weeks. Then a week with low training stress follows.

During the following sequence I begin the first week above the level of the previous sequence. I don't train at all the last week before the event, except for 1-2 short and relaxed training sessions at the start of the week.

This should enable my body to recover completely from the stress of training, and to perform at full capacity during the competition.

Super-Compensation

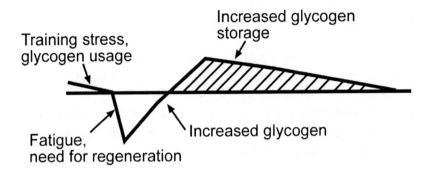

Super-Compensation is an increase in performance capacity brought about by placing stress on the body in training and allowing oneself to recover from it, with these processes taking place at correctly selected intervals.

After the stress of training is over, the body not only recoups its preparedness to attain the same performance level, but even makes possible a higher performance level for a certain time period.

If this higher performance level is used for each new training session, a continuous enhancement of performance results. If the time between training sessions is too great, the "training effect" is lost (A proper stimulation is achieved by training at least 3 times per week).

On the other hand, if you train too often the body doesn't have enough time to regenerate and the performance level goes down (over-training).

Targeted regeneration is thus just as important as training.

Mental Strength

To me, this term denotes qualities such as motivation, "stick-to-itiveness", will power, flexibility, ability to handle stress, etc.

The longer the competition you are participating in lasts and/or the more speed that is demanded of you, the more mental strength will decide whether you are successful or not.
If you want to finish a race that lasts 12, 24 or even more hours, you will have to train your mental strength as much as you train in the sport in which you are competing.

The absolute limit of your personal performance capacity in long races is much higher than you think.

But how can these performance reserves be made accessible in a competition?

How can you find out whether a physical limit has definitely been reached, or whether, for example, a motivation problem is behind it all?
You have to accept a real physical limit, and draw your own conclusions in a future training period and in an event you have selected.

The picture looks entirely different in the case of mental difficulties.
You won't get any advice like "You have a motivation problem" or "You could be faster".

Mental weaknesses make themselves known in a much more subtle manner. They show up, for example, in the way you deal with a competitive situation as far as your thoughts are concerned.

Should you content yourself with blaming it all on having a bad day, or can you activate mental and/or physical reserves in spite of the circumstances?

The good news first:

Normally mental strength increases as the training load increases.

The bad news:

Mental strength will only increase to the same extent as you consciously deal with the difficulties and blocks which are "presented" to you in training.
To put it in concrete terms: Your mental strength will grow only in so far as you take responsibility for a "deficit".

An example

I ran a long distance with a friend on a path that was new to him. In about the middle of the course, we ran back a short distance on the same path we had just covered.
As he perceived that he asked, having lost his motivation, "Are we really going to run back on the same path?"

Should he take part in a competition sometime which includes long, monotonous stretches, or in which several or many laps have to be run, the problem which had not been dealt with could quickly lead to an emotional low point; or, in the worst case, to dropping out of the event.

In concrete terms ...

If I can't get a good, suitable or helpful answer to a difficult problem arising in training, how and from where am I supposed to get an answer during a competitive event?

> **Then I need an answer which brings me up out of the depths, or encourages me to keep on going at a high performance level in long events!**

In training I also reflect over and over again on the way in which I motivate myself and how I deal with myself.

-- What kind of inner conversation do I carry on with myself in which training situations, and how do I pull myself out of a training crisis?

-- How do I handle unpleasant weather mentally?

-- What is triggered in me when I think about the next training unit of so and so many kilometers?

I give these internal processes a lot of attention, and I advise you urgently to do the same; for the repressed or unresolved problems which appear in training will, in all probability, make themselves known in a competition.

But there you have less desire and no leisure time to deal with this.

We haven't even begun to speak of the energy that is lost in this way, and it is precisely this energy that everyone needs so desperately in competition.

A further example

If you are not accustomed to (and find it unpleasant) training in pouring rain, strong wind and a temperature of 5 degrees (= 41 degrees Fahrenheit), such weather conditions could very well cause you to have a minor or major crisis in a competition (if you react like this often).

When something is unpleasant for me in training, I take a look at myself: Where do I have that from, and why am I of this persuasion?

On the topic of running in the rain:
Many people act as if it were the worst personal catastrophe to be struck by a raindrop.
Are they still hearing things that were told to them in their childhood, such as "You'll get sick -- you could get pneumonia!"?

Even when I got thoroughly soaked in the rain I stayed healthy, as long as I produced enough warmth by running. After a run like that, take a shower, put on warm clothes and everything will be fine.
It is especially important in an athletic competition not to be dependent upon external conditions (or, the less dependent you are, the better).

Being at odds with the weather, or worrying about how many spectators there are (or athletes) just robs you of energy. Rather, you should be focusing on internal processes. What should I drink, when should I eat something … .

During my 24-hour run (162k) children came to the running course after an hour, and one of them made fun of us:

"Ha! ha!, only 23 more hours!"

That was right, there were still 23 hours of running to go. The child did not swear at us or throw tomatoes, but I still allowed myself to become unmotivated for a minute.
This was due to my own feeling of insecurity and lack of experience, not knowing what would be coming my way for the next 23 hours.

When I let myself become distracted by inner processes (beliefs, internal dialog, memories) or external conditions, and lose my focus on the competition at hand, energy is dissipated without my noticing it.
Then it is not available to me, especially at low points. And in my 24-hour run there were quite a lot of low points to overcome -- as was the case with other runners, too. The long length of time, tiredness, a blister on the ball of the foot ... .

This applies to every training session as well, though on a smaller scale.

How do I improve my mental strength?

1. Perception of inner processes

-- Sense and accept that you have a certain conviction or feeling.

-- From where and why do you have a certain limiting belief?

-- Why do certain feelings like anger, fear or sadness surface in me?

2. Evaluate these internal processes and deal with the issues that are involved.

-- Learn a method that suits you and make regular use of it -- (meditation, relaxation exercises …).

3. Here and now

-- Concentrate on what you are doing in training and in competition. When I run, I concentrate on the next stride.

-- If I look too far ahead I could lose motivation if I see a steep climb or I could trip over a root.

-- If I think about whether I will still be fit in 10 hours it robs me of my energy. **Right now** there is no answer -- my brooding yields no result.
In the course of the competition I am sure to find out.

-- If I concern myself with what has already happened, it also will distract me.

It is important to be in the here and now in my perception (internal/external) and in what I am paying attention to.
Only in the present can I act and make decisions or utilize my energy in the most efficient manner in a competition.

It has been my experience that having this attitude in training enables me to train over long stretches effortlessly.
Sometimes during the first 20 minutes I haven't yet found the proper rhythm, but after that I feel great inner peace and enjoy the training session.

If you should consider participating in a competition that lasts 12, 24 or even more hours, then such inner peace will make things go much more easily for you in the event.

If you are just beginning to learn an endurance sport, this will be equally true for you. Only the distance will be different.

The mental challenges are always there -- whether you are a novice going 5k or are more advanced and attempting a 24-hour run.

4. Reflection

Take a regular look at past training or competition situations.

Physically: What was good?
What wasn't good?

Mentally: What was good?
What wasn't good?

The value of doing this is that you are learning with set goals in mind, and will be even better prepared for future training sessions and competitions, for the probability is very high that an unresolved issue will emerge.

When you are reflecting on past experiences (whether in daily life, training or competition) look carefully at the experience from the "beginning" to the "end". When I say "look at" I mean an honest examination -- don't minimize anything, or ignore a detail ... .

Rather: What was it **really** like?

For example:

-- What was the cause of the situation?

-- How did I react to it?

-- Were my actions appropriate and helpful ... ?

What should I change from here on out?

-- What did I learn that I can use in the future?

-- What do I need to learn as fast as possible?

-- What additional experiences do I require?

-- What resources can I activate?

Equipment (using running as an example)

Running shoes

If you are training regularly, I recommend that you buy the shoes in a specialty shop where you can view a video analysis.
Even though shoes may appear to be identical, the different brands and models will fit differently and affect your feet differently depending upon the anatomy of your feet.
Let the sales personnel help you to pick out the right shoes for you, regardless of brand or model.
By doing this, you will reduce the amount of stress placed on your entire body.
The "wrong" running shoe can lead to a change in body posture and to premature fatigue or abrasions.

Clothing

Pleasant running -- even when it is cold or wet -- is definitely possible with functional running apparel (made of synthetic materials). This enables moisture to be given off (sweat, rain). There is only a danger of catching a cold when the moisture is not carried off and the body cools down.

Forehead light

This is for running in the night or at dusk or dawn. A forehead light helps you to see obstacles (tree roots, stones, etc.) in time, but its primary value lies in the fact that others will be able to see you.

Pulse watch

If you are a novice runner, a pulse watch will help you to develop a feeling for the relationship between speed and pulse.
But a pulse watch is not really necessary. If you can converse fluently you are in Zone 1. If you must pause to catch your breath while conversing you are in Zone 2.

The advantage of a pulse watch for advanced athletes is that it will aid in determining the ideal training zones for improving performance.

One disadvantage of a pulse watch is that you can begin to forget to pay attention to your own physical needs (maybe it would be good for me to run faster today, but my pulse watch is going off again ...).
The training effect not only results from training at a certain heart rate, but also from your feeling well or other body reactions.
These can change from moment to moment.

Stretching Exercises

Repetitive motions which go on for a long period of time, and are typical of endurance sports, have two effects on the muscles involved:

-- Muscle endurance improves along with intramuscular coordination (the movements become easier and easier).

-- The muscles are strained in a one-sided manner by the similarity of the motions, and the opposing muscle reacts by shortening.

Shortened muscles have two significant disadvantages:

-- A shortened muscle provides less endurance.

-- A shortened muscle makes the work of its counterpart harder, and thus leads to increased strain and greater energy consumption.

For training this means that you should do your stretching exercises AFTER the training session, in order to balance off this one-sided stress; that is, to relax the muscles and tendons.

Well-stretched muscles support and improve stride length and rate when you are running. The result is a higher running velocity. Stretching exercises also relax the tendons utilized in running; and, in this way, reduce the risk of injury to the tendons.

The Most Important Stretching Exercises

Do not do these before a training session. This only increases the danger of injury.

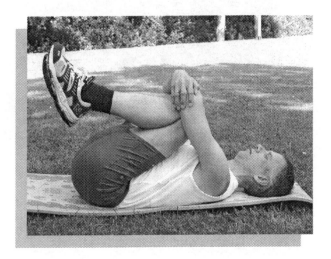

Lumbar spine

The back and neck lie stretched on the ground. Embrace both knees and pull them toward the body. Rock a little to the left and right.

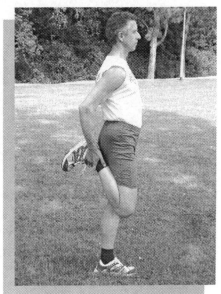

Front thigh musculature

Leave the knees at the same height.
Pull the heel up to the buttocks.
Then, switch sides.

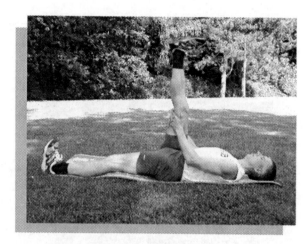

Rear thigh musculature

Lie flat on the back.
Hold the stretched leg vertically.
Then, switch sides.

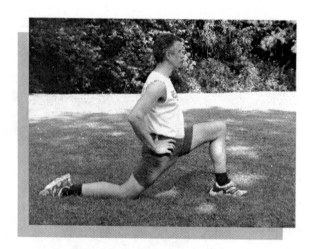

Hip benders / Psoas
The back and the left lower leg are
vertical. Push the pelvis slightly
toward the front. Then, switch sides.

Calves

Extend the rear leg.
Push the pelvis toward
the front until the
stretching of the calf
can be felt.
Then, switch sides.

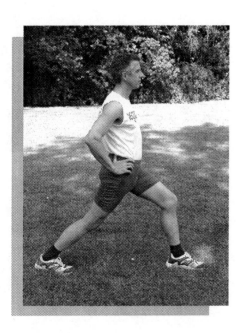

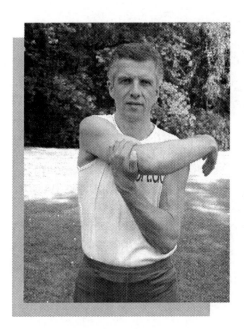

Shoulder blade /
back deltoid

Hold the arm at the
elbow at shoulder height
(about 20 cm = 8 inches
away from the body).
Pull the elbow diagonally to
the upper body toward the
left (see photo).
Then, switch sides.

Triceps

Hold the right upper
arm vertically, and
close the right hand
a little.
Pull the right elbow
slightly in the
direction of the head.
Then, switch sides.

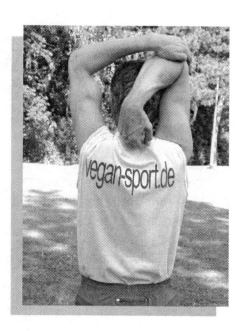

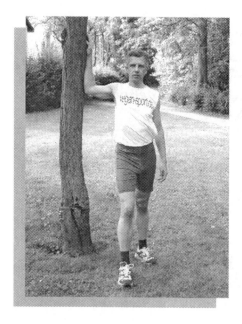

Front deltoid

Press the lower arm against
a wall or a tree (elbow at a
90 degree angle), keeping
the elbow at shoulder height.
Put the right foot in front of
the left foot.
Turn the upper body slowly
away from the tree.
Then, switch sides.

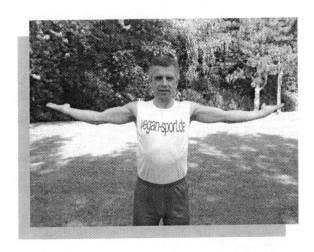

Biceps

Press the outstretched arms slowly to the rear at shoulder height (with the palms of the hands turned upward).

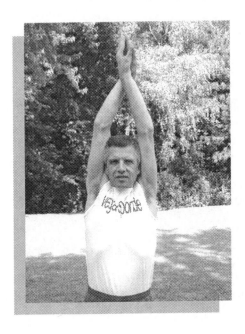

Latissimus / broad back muscle

Pull both arms up with crossed wrists (palms against each other).

Upper Body Exercises

As was already mentioned in the chapter **Running Style**, a strong trunk musculature supports running and swimming -- especially over longer stretches.

Therefore the strengthening of the trunk muscles should also be carried out in a targeted manner in endurance training.

A few examples of how the most important abdominal and back muscles can be trained:

Back musculature -- above all:
>   -- Broad back muscle
>   -- Trapezius muscle

Abdominal muscles -- above all:
>   -- External oblique abdominal muscle
>   -- Rectus abdominus
>   -- Internal oblique abdominal muscle

Novices
Depending on the exercise, hold it for 20 seconds or do 20 repetitions.

Advanced
Depending on the exercise, hold it for 30-60 seconds or do 40 repetitions.

A variation of this training is to perform the following exercises in the order listed, and then to do another round (or more).

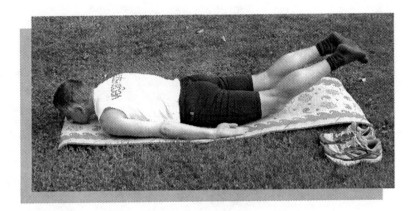

Procedure: Lie down on your stomach, and with both
legs stretched out, raise them up and hold
this position.

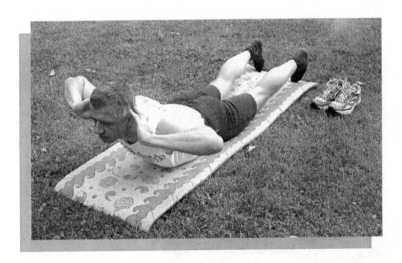

Procedure: Prone position, touch the ears with the hands
and raise the upper body (no hollow back);
hold.

203

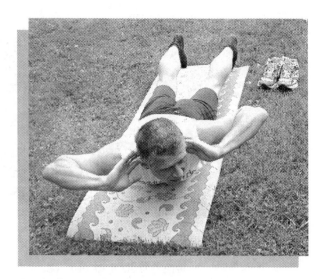

Procedure: Like the previous exercise, but turn
the upper body to the left and hold.

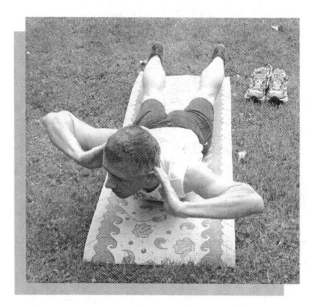

Procedure: Like the previous exercise, but turn to the right.

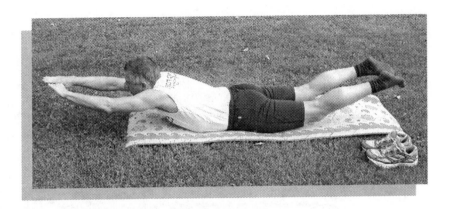

Procedure: Stretch out both arms and both legs and
lift them up at the same time. Hold.

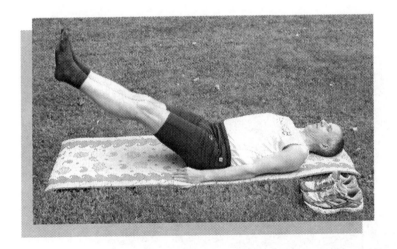

Procedure: Stretch out both legs and raise them simultaneously.
Hold. Don't use the arms for support -- it is the
abdominal muscles that are being trained.

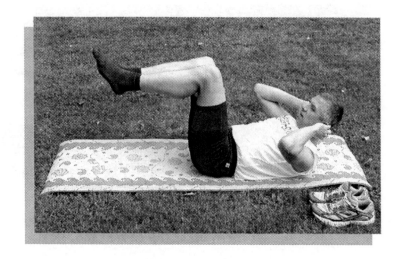

Procedure: Hold both legs at a 90 degree angle.
Place hands on ears and raise upper
body slightly. Hold.

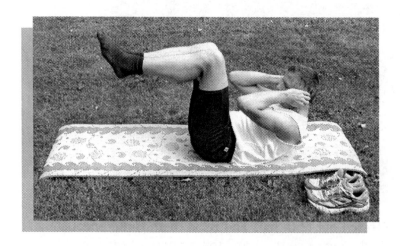

Procedure: Hold both legs at a 90 degree angle.
Place hands on ears and raise the upper
body several times as high as possible.

206

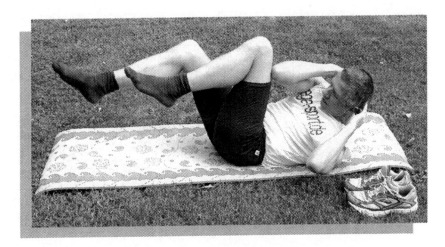

Procedure: Like the previous exercise. Raise the upper
body and touch the left leg with the right
elbow. Repeat several times.

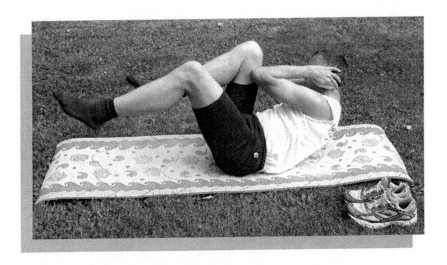

Procedure: Like the previous exercise. Raise the upper body
and touch the right leg with the left elbow.
Repeat several times.

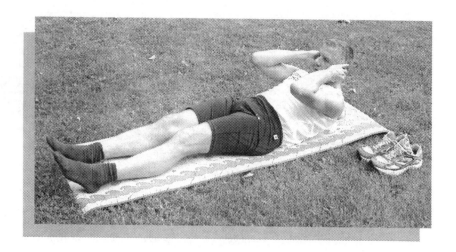

Procedure: The hands are touching the ears.
Raise upper body and hold.

Variation: Raise upper body several times.
Don't let the shoulders touch the
ground when lying back again.

Some concluding words . . .

When I have come to the end of a book, I ask myself some questions: "What new insights have I gained, which can I implement, and what changes will occur in my life because of this new knowledge?"

Therefore, I would like to stimulate you to ask yourself questions like those.

Some of what I have written might be new or unfamiliar to you. The **scientific and medical evidence** which establishes the relationship between the consumption of animal foodstuffs and the development of diseases is manifold and convincing.
The conclusions drawn from this always point in the same direction: The greater the intake of fruit and vegetables, the healthier a person is (Naturally, other factors need to be taken into consideration, such as exercise, smoking, stress, etc.).

There is much that speaks for making a decision to begin a balanced, varied **vegan diet**, for it provides ideal nourishment.

In the beginning phase it could very well be that the implementation of the new knowledge is not so easy. It is possible that old issues, such as self-defeating behaviors, feeling comfortable with an unhealthy life style or being accustomed to being overweight must be re-worked.

But you can rest assured that once you have the initial phase behind you, you will sense significant improvement in vitality, fitness and health.

I wish you great success and new vitality through vegan nutrition and endurance sports, in the beginning of your new dietary venture as well as in the many healthy years to come.

List of Sources

Source 1: Runner World 04/2005

Source 2: MDR, Sendung FAKT, 15.03.04

Source 3: ZDF, Sendung: Der Tod der Fische, 05.10.05

Source 4:http://www.fischen-tut-weh.de/Schmerz.html

Source 5: www.vegan.de

Source 6:
Ernährungsbericht 2004 der Bundesregierung ISBN   3-88749-183-1

Source 7:
http://www.vitaminwelten.com/index.php?id=218&tx_rlmpofficedocume
nts_pi1[showPage]=17&cHash=5ada463264#

Source 8:
The Comparative Anatomy of Eating von Dr. Milton R. Mills,
www.vegsource.com/veg_faq/comparative.htm
www.foodrevolution.org/askjohn/30.htm
www.peta.de/kampagnen/vegetarismus/natfood/physiologie.php
Neal Barnard, The Power of Your Plate, Book Publishing Company:
Summertown, Tenn., 1990, p. 170.

Source 9:
Schweizerische Herzstiftung,   www.swissheart.ch
PD Dr. Rubino Mordasini, Medienmitteilung 15.Juni 2004

Source 10:
Prof. Dr. Dr. h.c. mult. Harald zur Hausen, Vorsitzender und
wissenschaftliches Mitglied des Stiftungsvorstandes des Deutschen
Krebsforschungszentrums Heidelberg

Source 11:
Deutsches Institut für Ernährungsforschung Potsdam-Rehbrücke (DIFE),
Broschüre: Krebsprävention durch Ernährung www.dife.de
(Stiftung des öffentlichen Rechts und Mitglied der Wissenschafts-
gemeinschaft Gottfried Wilhelm Leibniz. Die Grundfinanzierung erhält die
Stiftung zu gleichen Teilen vom Land Brandenburg und vom Bund.)

Source 12:
Elizabeth Holly et al., Universität von Kalifornien, San Francisco -
www.ucsf.edu Cancer, Epidemiology, Biomarkers and Prevention,
September 2005, http://cebp.aacrjournals.org/
www.wissenschaft.de/wissen/news/257650.html

Source: 13: Prof. Walter J. Veith "Diet and Health", Medpharm 1998
Dr. Langley, Gill, Vegane Ernährung, Echo Verlag 1999
Lehrbücher der Inneren Medizin, z.B.: Herold "Innere Medizin", 2001
Lehrbücher der Pathologie (z.B.: Silbernagl, Lang "Taschenatlas der
Pathophysiologie" , Thieme Verlag 1998),   Zeitschrift CO'MED
Mikronährstofftherapie beim Kolonkarzinom, Ausgabe 8/2005

Source 13-1: Basiswissen Biochemie mit Pathobiochemie
ISBN 3-540-67389-X Seite 632,
http://www.netdoktor.de/krankheiten/fakta/gallensteine.htm

Source 14: McDougall, John A., M.D., and McDougall, Mary A., The
McDougall Plan, New Century Publishers, Inc., pp. 49-51

Source 15: Online-Magazin Profil.at
www.profil.at/?/articles/0524/560/114796.shtml

Source 16: http://de.wikipedia.org/wiki/Ballaststoff
http://www.nutrisun.at/gesundh.htm
http://www.gmf-info.de/Ballaststoffe.pdf

Source 16-1: http://de.wikipedia.org/wiki/Quinoa
http://www.nature.de/artikel/nahrung/descript/quinoa.htm

212

Source 17: Weltgesundheitsorganisation (WHO) - Bericht über Ernährung, Nahrung und Vorbeugung von chronischen Krankheiten. Genf, 1990

Source 18:
ADA Reports Position of the American Dietetic Association and Dietitians of Canada: Vegetarian diets doi:10.1053/jada.2003.50142
www.eatright.org   www.adajournal.org

Source 19: Sun Ha Jee und Kollegen, Yonsei-Universität in Seoul, Fachmagazin JAMA (Ausg. 293, Nr. 1, S. 194).
www.wissenschaft.de/wissen/news/248059.html

Source 20:   www.ironsport.de/Fette.htm
www.isarlauf.de/sportmedizin/ernaehrung/fett.htm

Source 21: Bundesforschungsanstalt für Ernährung Karlsruhe, Prof. Dr. J. F. Diehl Ltd. Dir. u. Prof. a. D., Prof. Dr. Gerhard Rechkemmer Leiter des Instituts für Ernährungsphysiologie der Bundesforschungsanstalt für Ernährung,   http://www.bfa-ernaehrung.de/Bfe-Deutsch/Information/e-docs/DiehlText.pdf

Source 22:
http://www.dge.de/modules.php?name=News&file=article&sid=475

Source 23:
Schweizerische Gesellschaft für Ernährung – www.sge-ssn.ch   TABULA – Zeitschrift für Ernährung, Ausgabe April 2004 ab Seite 4

Source 24: Antioxidantien-Studien:
1.: C.H. Hennekens et al: Lack of effect of long term supplementation with beta-carotene on the incidence of malignant neoplasms and cardiovascular disease. New England Journal of Medicine, 1996, 334, S.1145.
2.: The Alpha-Tocopherol, Beta Carotene Cancer Prevention Study Group: The effect of vitamin E and beta carotin an the incidence of lung cancer and other cancers in male smokers. New England Journal of Medicine, 1994, 330, S.1029.   3.: G.S. Omenn et al.: Effects of a combination of beta-carotene and vitamin A on lung cancer and cardiovascular disease. New England Journal of Medicine, 1996, 334, S.1150.

Source 25:
Zeitschrift CO'MED, Ausgabe 05/05, Calcium, Seite 4ff

Source 25-1:
http://www.webmed.ch/docs/L-Carnitin/L-Carnitin.htm
http://gin.uibk.ac.at/thema/sportundernaehrung/carnitin.html

Source 25-2:
Handbuch der Lebensmittelchemie, Bd 1
Die Bestandteile der Lebensmittel, S.167-307

Source 26:
Archives of Internal Medicine; vol. 165, pp. 1-6, March 28, 2005
http://mednews.wustl.edu/news/page/normal/4971.html

Source 27:
Medical hypotheses; VOL: 53 (6); p. 459-85 /199912/

Source 27-1:
 http://www.milchlos.de/milos_0406g.htm
http://www.aerztezeitung.de/docs/1998/01/28/016a0401.asp?cat=/me
dizin/krebs/prostatakrebs

Source 28:
Basiswissen Biochemie mit Pathobiochemie
ISBN 3-540-67389-X Seite 484f

Source 29:
Zeitschrift CO'MED, Ausgabe 05/05, Ernährungsproblem Nr.1: Adipositas,
Seite 12f,   Basiswissen Biochemie mit Pathobiochemie ISBN 3-540-
67389-X Seite 465f

Source 30:
ltd. Oberarzt Dr.med. Th.Müller, Main-Taunus-Kliniken Hofheim
3.Ärzte-Symposium Herz/Lunge, Sport und Gesundheit, 10.06.05 Kelheim

Source 31:

Priv.Doz.Dr.med. S.Blankenberg, Kardiologe, Oberarzt der II.Medizinischen Klinik, Johannes Gutenberg-Universität Mainz

3.Ärzte-Symposium Herz/Lunge, Sport und Gesundheit, 10.06.05 Kelheim

Source 32:

Deutsches Medizin-Netz , Nürnberg

www.medizin-netz.de/framesets/fseticentertrinken.htm

Gatorade Sports Science Institute, Barrington, Illinois

www.gssiweb-de.com/reflib/refs/25/SSEroundtable_43_deutsch.cfm

Gesundheitsinformationsnetz GIN, Institut für Biostatistik und Dokumentation der Medizinischen Universität Innsbruck Trinken im Sport

Dr. Kurt A. Moosburger, Facharzt für Innere Medizin und Sportarzt

Further Reading

natural eating   ISBN 3-89530-064-0

Durch Mineralien zu Wohlbefinden und Leistungskraft   3-7742-1489-1

Mineralien das Erfolgsprogramm   ISBN 3-453-86928-1

Ernährungsbericht 2004 der Bundesregierung ISBN: 3-88749-183-1

Prof. Walter J. Veith Diet and Health, Medpharm 1998

Dr. Langley, Gill, Vegane Ernährung, Echo Verlag 1999

Lehrbücher der Inneren Medizin, z.B.: Herold Innere Medizin, 2001

Lehrbücher der Pathologie (z.B.: Silbernagl, Lang "Taschenatlas der Pathophysiologie", Thieme Verlag 1998)

www.channing.harvard.edu/nhs/history/index.shtml#histI

Chapter Dietary Supplementation, Methods of Analysis, the Analysis of Nutritional Needs:

Naturheilpraxis für Körper und Geist   Petra Wiegand, Heilpraktikerin Hornauer Straße 174, D - 65779 Kelkheim

Telefon 06195 – 67 69 39 www.wiegand-naturheilpraxis.de

Lightning Source UK Ltd.
Milton Keynes UK
UKOW022037050213

205859UK00004B/120/A